OVERCOMING IMPOTENCE

MARY WILLIAMS grew up in Hampshire and London, where she was a student teacher in the 1960s and where she met her husband. They moved to Lancashire, and have three adult sons and a foster son. She trained with Relate in marital and psychosexual therapy and later worked with children and families for the NSPCC and the Health Service. She recently retired from her post as staff counsellor at a university to take up writing full time, and has published poetry, short stories and a collection of humorous anecdotes about local life. She is the author of *Make Up or Break Up? Making the Most of Your Marriage*, also published by Sheldon Press.

D1099634

Overcoming Common Problems Series

A full list of titles is available from Sheldon Press,
1 Marylebone Road, London NW1 4DU, and on our website at
www.sheldonpress.co.uk

Overcoming Common Problems Series

Overcoming Common Problems Series

Overcoming Common Problems

Overcoming Impotence

Mary Williams

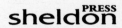

First published in Great Britain in 2003 by
Sheldon Press
1 Marylebone Road
London NW1 4DU

British Library Cataloguing-in-Publication Data

A catalogue record for this book is available from the British Library

ISBN 0–85969–905–6

1 3 5 7 9 10 8 6 4 2

Typeset by Deltatype Limited, Birkenhead, Merseyside
Printed in Great Britain by Biddles Ltd
www.biddles.co.uk

Contents

I would like to acknowledge thanks to Meg and Vicky for their invaluable insights and opinions. They know who they are!

Introduction

Impotence is a sensitive, touchy subject. Nowadays it is more often referred to as 'erectile dysfunction', a broader term, but scarcely more palatable. What does the word 'impotence' suggest to you? The dictionary defines it as 'wanting in physical, intellectual, or moral power; of the male, lacking the power of sexual intercourse'. This definition omits the overwhelming sense of frustration, embarrassment and powerlessness the word also contains. This applies to both men and their partners. The dictionary provides us with other words too: 'inefficiency', 'incapacity', 'emasculation' and 'disarmed', 'inoperative', 'inadequate', 'powerless'. We need to separate these associations from the real physical state of erectile dysfunction. How can we undo this damaging perception of what is, for many men at some time in their lives, a normal state?

For me, the negative words I have heard people associate with impotence are often not those above, but rather 'tired', 'weary', 'upset', 'angry', 'dispirited', 'fed up', 'lacking in desire or confidence'. A debate is beginning now, I believe, which is not unlike the past debate around female breast cancer. There is now more open discussion and less embarrassment about revealing that one has had breast cancer, and a sense of the issue being 'normalized', which is helpful for women who wish to share their experiences. I believe we are at the beginning of a change in attitude towards impotence too, and that this most sensitive of subjects will become less of a taboo subject for men to talk about, if they wish to do so.

I would like to return to the physical reality of the sexual state of impotence. It means simply not being able, on more than 25 per cent of occasions, to get and maintain an erection sufficient for sexual intercourse. The man may want to feel aroused but not have an erection, or get one but lose it before intercourse or ejaculation. Or he may get an erection that is not firm enough for penetration. The cause may be organic, to do with illness, fatigue, age or medication, or psychological, or a mixture of both. Interestingly, several textbooks which assert that male impotence has in the majority of

1

cases an organic rather than a psychological origin, list depression as a medical factor causing impotence, along with other culprits such as diabetes and cardio-vascular disease. So whether you regard depression as a psychological or a physical cause of impotence appears to affect how the statistics are collated. What does not seem to be in dispute, however, is that depression and impotence often go hand in hand; the lifting of depression frees up the *joie de vivre*, and the flow of energy, both physical, intellectual and sexual, is increased. Depression is exhausting and deadening, and leaves us with a view of the world that is grey, pointless and uninspired. More of this later.

It seems very important in any discussion of impotence to make a distinction between loss of desire and loss of function. It's normal for men experiencing depression, stress or great disappointment to be temporarily uninterested in sex. It's the least of their concerns. However, if you are a person who expects to be able to perform no matter what, and who doesn't make the link between mind and body, the fact that your body will not obey you and create an erection to order will be quite a shock. It may seem as if this is yet one more thing that has gone wrong, and because it's an obvious and visible difficulty, the lack of an erection can easily become the focus of the problem, when in fact it may be a side-effect, righting itself as soon as the emotional equilibrium is restored. A number of men will not want to hear this, however, and I would like to invite any men reading this to keep an open mind and to ask themselves the question: 'Am I reasonably relaxed, happy and contented?' before heading for the Viagra clinic or trying other expensive, quick-fix solutions. Of course, it's necessary to have a medical check-up, if problems persist, to exclude obvious physical reasons, but your GP is more likely to prescribe an antidepressant, if he suspects your impotence is caused by depression, than he is Viagra. There is a chicken-and-egg question to be answered here, of course, as impotence can cause depression as well as result from it.

If you are a person who likes to look for solutions to problems on the Internet, you will find a great many websites selling Viagra and other medications. This is because Viagra is generally not available on free NHS prescription except to certain defined categories of patients. Your GP may well be able to give you a private prescription, but it isn't cheap. Selling this and other similar drugs is consequently a major industry and a cynic might suggest that they are promoted to the exclusion of other, more holistic and gentle approaches. It is vitally important, if you wish to use Viagra, that you are not taking nitrate medication for angina, as the outcome could be fatal. This is why it is best to obtain a doctor's prescription and advice rather than attempt to do it yourself. We'll look more carefully at Viagra in Chapter 2.

If the answer to that first question you asked yourself was 'No', you may want to ask yourself the second question: 'What changes have there been in my life recently, and have I allowed myself to process them fully?' By processing, I mean allowing time to adjust, think about, and experience the feelings associated with the event, whether it's a bereavement, loss of a job, a birthday with a zero at the end of it, a health problem or general stress. If the answer to the first question was 'No', there may be other issues to sort out before your potency can return to its normal state. If you regard yourself as happy, satisfied and content in the main with your relationship and life, but are troubled by recurring impotence, and a medical check excludes organic illness, there are other helpful courses open to you. We will look at different options later in this book.

Impotence is a shared problem. It affects both of you, yet often it seems that the male takes total responsibility for what he perceives as his failure. I would like to challenge this assumption. You may feel you are protecting your partner by trying to stay in control of it all, but she will undoubtedly feel differently about it and possibly be slightly annoyed at being excluded from what is also her relationship. She may, of course, also blame you, or herself, for not finding her sufficiently attractive, and in this respect it becomes very much her problem too. Impotence is rarely to do with physical attractiveness alone, though big physical changes may create their own problems.

Part of the problem in our perception of impotence lies within the symbolic aspect of the sexual act and the way in which males think about themselves as sexual people. The self-esteem and confidence they have in their everyday lives is tied in with this perception. It may be sometimes harder for the man to cope with a wider sense of failure, such as the loss of a job, than the failure to maintain an erection from time to time. For many men, performance is all, whether it's at work or at home, and they understandably like to feel in control of it.

INTRODUCTION

The sex act is, by its very nature and history, an aggressive act. The female partner receives the penis, it enters her; the man penetrates her with his penis. One enters the other, and testosterone-fuelled erections enable this to happen. The words associated with this activity are strong, masculine words – 'hard-on', 'thrust', 'penetrate', 'erect', 'impregnate', 'ejaculate'. If a woman does not always have an orgasm, or sometimes does not even get aroused, it is unlikely to cause a major upset between the couple. The female will be most likely to acknowledge to herself that she is overtired, unwell or simply not in the mood, and there's an end to it. Not so the anxious male. His masculinity is under question; he feels a failure, no matter what his partner says or does. His concept of himself as a potent male has taken a battering and the next time he attempts to have intercourse he may wonder if it will happen again. Wondering generates anxiety and doubt and so the cycle is continued. A man in tune with himself and his partner may realize that he is lacking in desire and energy from time to time, that he is feeling 'temporarily indisposed', to use an old-fashioned expression, and not place demands on himself that his body cannot meet. If he can express this to his partner, so much the better. She'll know then that it isn't her he feels negative about, it's just that he's not in the mood. If he ignores his inner self he may find, when he tries to have a sexual encounter, that his body isn't interested. This will be very alarming for him if it's never happened before and consequently he will be filled with gloom. A repeated failure will endorse and give weight to this feeling. Having felt depressed before, but not admitted it, he feels even worse now. This is a situation he feels he has to fix, and quickly. His penis and its disobedience become the centre of his attention, and the other events in his life that have temporarily depleted him of his energy, sexual drive and potency, will not be dealt with. This is a great pity.

There are, as we will see, many causes of male impotence. Drugs companies, knowing that they're on to a good thing, tend, in my opinion, to overplay the medical factors in order to sell their products, but in fact the truth is that it's often a combination of factors which have the cumulative effect of undermining the confidence of the male to get and maintain his erection. Just as nothing succeeds like success, nothing fails so much as repeated failure. This book sets out to explore all these factors and to look

4

objectively at some of the different treatments on offer for impotence with a medical and physical basis, and the different triggers and factors in maintaining the psychological aspects of the problem. We will also consider the effects of impotence on a partnership and marriage, and explore some of the hidden agendas that may exist in these relationships, in which the distress of the female partner is sometimes ignored by those working with the male partner alone.

There are many marriages that incorporate episodes of impotence with barely a hiccough, others that manage less well, still others where the impotence of the male is of benefit to his partner in some way and maintained by mutual consent. Understanding the relationship between the two spouses is crucial to the work of the sex therapist, as without the wholehearted co-operation of the spouse any treatment programme is unlikely to succeed over time. The wife or female partner is the therapist's right-hand woman. We will look into this more closely later in the book.

It is estimated that in the United States alone, over three million men are impotent at any one time. Most men over the age of 45 experience impotence from time to time. Looking at these statistics a different way, this also means that most older men do *not* experience impotence most of the time; it is very often an intermittent or transient state, often caused by external factors and the health or tiredness of the partners.

The biggest factor preventing people obtaining help, whether from an outside agency or a partner, is embarrassment followed by shame. Even more humiliating than not getting and maintaining an erection, for which there may be a physical reason, is the failure to cope with your life and to be a real man (whatever that is perceived as being). The admission that you are depressed is a hard one to make and for a number of men this is a real sticking point.

Permission to talk about this problem helps. Giving yourself permission is the first step. A sensitive doctor, nurse, psychiatrist or other source of help should not shy away from the subject, but it can be helpful to have more direct permission from them to talk about it. If your doctor asks: 'And how are things between you and your wife?' when you report back after a prostatectomy, it's permission, but even clearer would be him asking: 'Any problems with your love life?' Doctors vary a great deal in how happy (or not) they feel about asking personal questions of their patients. I have only ever been asked once by a doctor how my sex life was now with my husband, since the difficult birth of our baby, and the question was put in such a way and with such gentle concern that I immediately confessed all and was grateful that a difficult subject had been broached. I hope to dispel some of this embarrassment in the following chapters.

One of the male figures in modern literature to have experienced impotence from time to time and not attached any great importance to it is the heroine's lover in Erica Jong's *Fear of Flying*. The heroine is interested in him partly because he does not attach huge importance to maintaining his erections, but also because he is very appreciative of her larger than average bottom and more than willing to make love in ways that give her pleasure, rather than solely depending on his penis. On a similar theme, in his best-selling work *Men and Sex*, Bernie Zilbergeld headed one chapter in a way that made men who read it laugh aloud. It was headed 'Twelve Feet Long and Made of Steel'. It debunked the self-imposed myth of the super-phallus and male performance and allowed males to view the subject with humour and self-forgiveness in a way that was refreshingly honest and down to earth. My hope is that this work will contribute to this debate in a way that gives food for thought alongside practical information and some evaluation of treatments, and that the wives or partners of men experiencing erectile problems will also gain some comfort from reading it.

1

The physiology of impotence

In this book, I have used sexual words that have a neutral value and are generally accepted as medically correct, but at the same time I am well aware that many people do not think of their own sexual organs in these terms. It's what they tell the doctor about if they're trying to be polite. But sometimes a person may not know the 'correct' terminology for the problem, or find the words for it difficult to use. After all, there's a difference between saying, 'I can't get it up,' and 'I can't get an erection'. Doctors, especially if their first language isn't English or they are not aware of local euphemisms, may not comprehend when told that a female 'front bottom' is sore, or the 'old man's not working', but the patient may be highly embarrassed to use the word 'vagina' or to say that he can't get an erection, because these words seem more exposing and serious.

Consequently, I feel it is important for couples to discover what their own language is, and what they feel comfortable with. In the North West, the word 'flower' is a euphemism for female genitalia, in other parts of the country 'flower' would not be recognized. In London girls used to be told to 'keep your hand on your ha'penny', whereas in Lancashire it's 'tuppence'. In Urdu the child's word for a penis is the same as that for a small red chilli, and there are other euphemisms for genital parts in every language. These words are often thought of as 'dirty' but actually in the main they are not words used in a pejorative sense as swear words, but simply as descriptive language, albeit with a vulgar edge at times. The pejorative, aggressive words are the kind of words that you hear if someone makes an obscene phone call to you, wants to express their displeasure by swearing, or wishes to shock or cause offence. Lovers sometimes use these words between themselves as part of their arousal pattern, but generally they are not public words.

So with this in mind, let's look at getting a *hard-on*, a *stiffie*, and *getting it up*, and the construction of the *willy, wedding tackle, old man, john thomas*, or the *crown jewels, cock, dick* or *knob*, followed by *having it off, giving her one, parking the Palethorpe* (after

7

Palethorpe's sausages), *fucking* and *making love*. These words (and hundreds more) express more exactly the intimate sexual activity of the couple than the neutral 'sexual intercourse', 'erection' or 'penis', but these are the words that are generally acceptable and so will be used in this book. If you and your partner are finding communication about sexual matters difficult, try having a competition to see who can write down the most words for each of the sexual parts, masturbation and intercourse. Then take it in turns to read aloud from your list and score one for every word or phrase shared, two for one your partner hasn't got. Have a prize ready for the winner, and have fun!

Now back to the mechanics.

Sexual drive and erections

We normally think of sexual drive and the ability to have erections as one and the same thing, but they're not. Sexual drive and libido are driven by testosterone, which is manufactured in the testes. This is the male hormone, responsible for the male characteristics of muscular strength, deeper voice, hairiness, aggression, and so on. But a man can have plenty of testosterone and not have erections. To have desire and drive but not the means of fulfilling them is the most frustrating of situations. Younger men who present with impotence are often in this category.

Conversely, a man may produce almost no testosterone yet have erections. He may have ability but no desire. And both desire, libido and erectile function can be switched off by psychological and physical events.

For the majority of men, desire, arousal and erection tend to follow on in sequence, whether they have slightly low testosterone or not. In situations where there is impotence something happens to interfere with this sequence.

Desire and arousal

We could say that desire is the feeling, arousal the manifestation of that feeling. Arousal begins with a stimulus. This can be:

• through sight (a glimpse of the partner's breasts, for example, or an erotic film or magazine);

8

- through hearing (a partner phoning you and expressing a sexual wish, a couple making love noisily in the next room);
- through smell (her perfume, sweat, hair); human sex hormones have a highly arousing smell;
- through touch (she brushes up against him, they kiss in an intimate way);
- through sexual thoughts or memories triggered by a situation (he remembers the last time she wore that dress).

Sexual arousal is highly conditionable, and each man will have his own personal triggers. Arousal, especially in young men, may happen a number of times in one day, and often cannot be acted upon, though the cumulative pressure of repeated arousal without ejaculation will lead to a need for either intercourse, masturbation or a sexual dream in which ejaculation occurs. This is because there is nowhere for semen to go in fit young men but out, and when the seminal vesicles (sperm stores) are full, an ejaculation takes care of the overflow. This is the same for men who have had a vasectomy, as the sperm is only a tiny percentage of the ejaculate and the remainder is seminal fluid. The sperm in this case is absorbed back into the body.

Erection

So what happens when a man has an erection? The sexual stimulus received by the brain triggers an increased blood supply to the penis, which swells and stiffens and begins to become erect. If there is no prospect of a full sexual act, the erection will subside; if sex is on the cards the erection becomes hard and firm.

While we're on the subject, an average length for a penis which isn't erect is between three and four inches, and smaller penises enlarge more than larger ones when erect. Having studied with interest many photographs of penises in both flaccid and erect states, I can safely state that there isn't *that* much difference in size between one erect penis and another; the difference is mainly visible between the flaccid ones, and flaccid small penises enlarge more when erect than do larger ones, which may thicken but not lengthen. Most heterosexual males don't get to look at other men when they are erect, so there is a certain false mythology around size, based on the flaccid state.

The blood is pumped into three sponge-like tubes, two either side of the third and main one, which forms the head of the penis and the urethra. These three spongy tubes fill up with blood and become engorged, and the foreskin, if the man has one, is pulled back over the glans, or head of the penis, to expose the glans. The scrotum changes its position too and moves away from the body a little in readiness. The scrotum begins to operate a hydraulic system to transport the sperm and the fluid it sits in along the vas deferens to the storage space by the bladder, from where it is ejaculated out via the urethra, by a series of muscular contractions. The common words for the ejaculated sperm are *spunk, jissom* and *come*. The erection can remain firm in many men for some time, but may wax and wane slightly as the amount of stimulation increases or decreases. At the point when ejaculation is almost inevitable, clear liquid will travel down the urethra and act as a cleansing and lubricating agent for the passage of sperm. As the urethra is also used for passing urine, this is necessary. Ejaculation usually happens soon after this, in a series of spasms, which push the sperm and fluid out of the body with some force. Almost as soon as this happens the blood starts to drain away from the penis and surrounding area and the erection subsides. There is then usually a sense of well-being and a relief of sexual tension. All this can happen with and without a partner.

What happens when the erection isn't there?

If a man experiences impotence, something happens to disturb this sequence. His body may refuse to obey the normal triggers and be inhibited from becoming aroused. He may simply not be interested, but thinks he should be. He may become aroused; then switch off without consciously wanting to. He may become partially erect, but not hard enough to enter his partner. There can be a number of physical as well as psychological reasons for this. Whatever the reason, a thorough assessment is usually helpful in discovering the cause. We will look into this in Chapter 2.

Night-time erections

Very important in the assessment of men experiencing impotence is to know whether they have night-time or early morning erections. Most men have erections or part-erections while they sleep; often they wake with them. If your doctor or therapist asks you and you're not sure, there are ways to find out. One way used to be sticking a strip of gummed paper around the penis and seeing if it had broken in the morning, though there are more sophisticated tests now. The partner can sometimes offer an opinion too, but often the man will be aware of night-time erections. If a man has night-time erections or can stimulate himself on his own with no difficulty, the problem is generally within his relationship and his own confidence. Or he's just depressed. He knows there's nothing wrong with the plumbing.

If a man *never* has an erection, on his own, at night, or with his partner, it's safe to say there is likely to be a physical cause for the condition, though his desire may remain strong. However, even when there is some physical impairment, there may be times when an erection is possible and it's on these occasions that intercourse can happen.

Primary impotence

Very rarely a man will never have had an erection followed by ejaculation. It's extremely rare, but if a man has a very tight or split foreskin, for example, the pain of erection will have inhibited him from sexual arousal. Very strict religious beliefs accompanied by punishment may also have a similar effect. The adverse conditioning in these men is very strong, and overcoming the associated fear and pain is a real challenge.

The woman's needs

Of course, in all of the above we are concentrating on the man and his arousal and erection. What about the woman? Without going into the physiological details of female arousal, disappointment and decreased confidence are sometimes the emotional consequence if the woman is left 'high and dry' time after time. She is likely to feel a failure, unattractive and unsuccessful if her man cannot get an erection and keep it when he is with her. After all, she must be doing something to put him off, especially if he remains concerned only about his own erection, or lack of it, and doesn't continue to make love to her in other ways. She may become resigned to not having a sex life with her husband and switch off her sexual feelings, fearing disappointment if she begins again. Often anger builds up, especially if the woman has a negative view of herself and her body, or her desirability. A woman with previous partners who have undermined her sexuality with critical or negative comments, or who have denigrated her in other ways, may be especially sensitive to the failure of the present partner to put this right. It is also true that many women are reluctant to give sexual pleasure and release to themselves, by masturbating, which puts all the responsibility and blame on to the man for their sexual and emotional satisfaction. This is neither fair nor likely to be of help.

But women, too, have sexual needs, and if their partner develops a real fear of failure, he may not want to put himself to the test with his partner. In giving some sexual satisfaction to his partner in other ways he is further reminded that this feast is something he cannot fully partake of. The woman can feel exposed and selfish in enjoyment of her own sexual arousal when her husband cannot take part more fully and gain the same satisfaction. All kinds of emotional inhibitors come into play here. Of these, hidden anger or guilt is very important, and couples in therapy will generally face a period of uncomfortable soul-searching to uncover these factors. For many males, unused to associating the psychological effects of impotence with the practical ones, this may be a disappointment, which is why, I suspect, the patent cures for impotence seem so appealing. It's much simpler to believe that there is a medical problem that needs treating than to investigate the relationship and the state of mind of you and your partner. Yet if there is medical intervention and no assessment of the overall state of the couple's relationship and emotional life, the medical intervention stands far less chance of working. Even with Viagra, or the newer drug, Uprima, you need a willing partner there to take part, if intercourse is to happen. Both these drugs work only in response to sexual stimulation. This is where the role of the partner is so important, as it may take more than the mere presence of a willing partner to provide the stimulation required. Some female partners find the use of other visual material, for example, hard to cope with, and this in itself can create problems.

12

Ruth and Andrew, a couple in their fifties, came to their local clinic for help because Andrew, after a spell of working much too hard, had begun to be impotent. He had been checked out by his doctor, who had given him some testosterone tablets, but they had made no difference to his sexual performance, though they improved his sense of general well-being. Ruth was the more forceful partner, very anxious to do the correct thing, and although an attractive woman appeared to have doubts about her appearance which her husband was very quick to dispel. Andrew, on the other hand, was very easy-going and rather passive and seemed older than he was. He was distressed at what he saw as his failure to have sex with his wife.

After a lengthy treatment programme of slow gradual increases in intimacy with no intercourse, his erections came back. Ruth and Andrew were very compliant with the demands of the programme, but the therapist felt that something was not quite right between them. At the end of treatment Andrew was fully functional and experienced full erections on the majority of occasions. Three months later they were sent individual evaluations, and hers was poor while his was excellent. Later she attended a clinic on her own and confessed that she had wanted to leave Andrew before he became impotent because he was so passive and unexciting. She had been unable to cope with the changes in him and the demands it placed on her. She felt she had done her duty in attending the clinic with him and complying with the programme, but secretly she did not want things to change.

This story, although true, is unusual, and is not intended as an awful warning to men experiencing temporary impotence – far from it. But it does highlight the tricky nature of relationships where sex is concerned.

Changes in the relationship

Because of the role of the partner and the fear of sexual failure for both, the therapist needs to ask the question 'How will this relationship change if this bit is fixed?' A marital and sexual relationship is a system. If one bit is altered, other bits have to change. Keeping pace with these other agendas and changes is vital for successful therapy. We will look at these issues more closely later in this book.

A couple, who we will call Maureen and Ken, made an appointment for Ken to see his doctor because he was getting infrequent erections which didn't last long enough for penetration. Maureen was more sexually experienced than Ken, having had many more partners, but sex between Maureen and Ken had been exciting and fun when they first got together. Ken's doctor checked his health and found nothing wrong.

He was prescribed Viagra and they used this a number of times with varying degrees of success. However, Maureen did not like the idea that their sex life depended on a medical remedy. Why was she unable to turn him on? What was wrong with her? It turned out that Maureen's ex-partners, who had been quite aggressive people, had left her feeling very inadequate in many ways, and she very much needed this present relationship to work in order to restore her self-esteem. Ken was not aggressive, though he could be verbally cruel at times. However, the person who was expressing the inadequacy was Ken who, being inexperienced, thought he was the cause of the problem. He did not want to compare himself to his wife's past lovers, but he suspected he didn't measure up. A few hurtful remarks about this, as in 'I'm sorry if I don't come up to scratch,' and 'I know this isn't what you're used to,' drove a wedge between them. They did have a deep love for one another however, and once some of this was out in the open and discussed and the couple had had a chance to be together on holiday away from the setting associated with failure, the problem quickly resolved.

Unlike the previous couple, there was nothing hidden going on in the relationship that they could not eventually discuss and resolve, and as they did so their relationship gained in trust and confidence.

Ambivalence

There is sometimes a deep ambivalence in both partners to engage in satisfying sex. The man's arousal may be squashed by the thought or feeling, 'I'm not going to set myself up for further humiliation,' and 'I want sex, but I don't want her, right now.'

This is because there is often hidden unexpressed anger or anxiety, which the partners have not dealt with. The female partner may not enjoy sexual activity with her partner very much, but may go along with it to please him or to avoid a row. Sooner or later her ambivalence will show itself and his body may respond with impotence. This was the case with Ruth and Andrew, mentioned earlier in this chapter.

2

Medical factors

There are several main medical causes of impotence that a doctor will want to investigate in a patient. The main one of these in younger men is diabetes, which if poorly managed can lead to damage in the nerve endings, and in older men hardening of the arteries decreases blood flow and can result in erectile difficulties. However, most men are aware that intermittent impotence can be one effect of diabetes, and it's hard to say whether the psychological impact of this information isn't, in fact, as damaging as the condition itself. Some studies suggest that the fear of impotence in some men is so great that it creates the condition. Many men who have diabetes have frequent maintained erections and enjoy a satisfactory sex life, taking in their stride the occasional time when it doesn't happen, and are relaxed about it. Those who are not confident in their relationship, or have a need to perform sexually to please a partner and who are more anxious generally, usually fare less well, especially if they do not manage their diabetes properly. One of the early signs of diabetes is ejaculation internally for the man, whose sperm may be discharged into his bladder. Any man experiencing orgasm without ejaculation for the first time should see his doctor. For couples anxious to have children, there are techniques for retrieving sperm and using it, despite this, and impotence need not feature at all.

For older men with hardening of the arteries, there are various drugs that may improve matters, but prevention is the best cure. Not smoking, a diet containing some fish oils and plenty of fruit and vegetable fibre, and regular exercise all help to maintain healthy circulation. Sexual activity is in itself good for you, whether it's alone or with a partner, as it keeps the genitals in working order and maintains the circulation. Here the old adage 'Use it or lose it' seems to apply.

A percentage of men who find it less and less possible to get or maintain an erection, as a result of peripheral nerve damage due to diabetes, or hardening of the arteries, will need further assistance to manage their sexual life. We will consider these other options separately later in this book.

Other conditions, including the most common one, hardening of the arteries, often exacerbated by smoking, and the more chronic illnesses such as Parkinson's, multiple sclerosis and other diseases of the nervous system, can also result in intermittent or regular erection difficulties. Doctors are well aware of this, but my advice would be not to anticipate it, but to enjoy what you do have while you have it.

Effects of medication

Another cause of male impotence is the side-effect of some drugs for the treatment of hypertension. Beta-blockers have long been implicated in impotence, but there are newer, less problematic drugs on the market today that do not have this effect. It is worth asking your doctor to change the drug to a different brand if you are on beta-blockers and think they are causing erection problems.

Because an erection needs blood to maintain it, any serious disturbance to the general circulation of blood in the body can impact on the sexual function. Arterial disease and blockages in major arteries do cause impaired blood flow to the penis, though a heart attack may have more of a psychological effect on the man, as fear of exertion and depression are great inhibitory factors.

Other drugs used in the treatment of some major illnesses, including mental illness, may also cause impotence. Chlorproma-zine-based drugs as well as imiprimine and amitriptyline are implicated here. If you are on such medication and suspect it may be causing impotence, or decreased sexual desire, you might find it useful to refer to a drug guide such as the BMA handbook, which will tell you exactly what the drug you are taking contains, and its effects. The direct NHS helplines will also offer information on this. Drugs change all the time as new preparations become available, and it's important to get up-to-date information from your doctor or from a recognized source, such as a health helpline, if you want to investigate your medication.

Many doctors test their patients for low testosterone levels, but it is very doubtful whether lowered testosterone *per se* has much of an impact on sexual performance, though it seems to enhance general well-being. Eunuchs who guarded the harems of eastern potentates were without testicles (and therefore testosterone) yet they could have erections. What they could not do was father children. Many men with decreased levels of the hormone are not impotent, and for those that are, the psychological effects of the drug, if administered, may make the difference. Diseases of the hormone or endocrine system can also result in impotence, though successful treatment can restore the sexual function in some cases. Doctors are reluctant to prescribe testosterone over a long period of time to men without endocrine disorders because of the effects on the body's own natural testosterone production, which may lessen.

Smoking

Another factor implicated in the onset of impotence, and which is less discussed, is smoking. Smoking causes peripheral nerve damage eventually, but even in the short term it decreases the flow of blood to the penis from the artery and also allows the blood to run off more quickly via the veins, so that getting and maintaining an erection becomes difficult. This effect is reversible up to a point, if the person gives up or cuts down their nicotine intake, and this can be a great incentive to giving up smoking! The longer-term damage to veins and arteries from the effects of smoking cannot be undone.

Chronic illness

Impotence may also be a symptom in severe kidney disease or multiple sclerosis (where it is often intermittent) and may also follow on from surgery for bowel problems, where the nerves have been damaged in surgery. For anyone experiencing impotence as a result of illness or surgery, there are a number of useful gadgets and gizmos that can help. Looked on as friendly toys or helpful adjuncts (in the way a vibrator may be for a woman), with a willing partner and a relaxed attitude, these can be most helpful. If the partner has nearly lost her life companion as a result of the illness causing his impotence, she may be afraid to embark on a renewed sexual life with him for fear of him hurting himself, and there will need to be some serious discussion about the impact of the illness on the emotional life of the couple, as part of the adjustment process. The system has to accommodate this new, difficult aspect of their life together. Use of a prosthetic device, in conjunction with friendly and appropriate therapeutic input for both partners, can be very helpful.

Spinal injuries

Men who have experienced a spinal injury can often become aroused in response to manual stimulation and may or may not ejaculate. Their response often depends on how great the damage to the spinal cord is, and whether it is high up or low down the spinal column. For a great many spine-injured men intercourse is possible and impotence is not a problem, though the mechanics of sexual intercourse may need some creative assistance. The same is true for people with cerebral palsy, spina bifida and other similar conditions. All cases are individual and need to be individually assessed, but in general the attitude of others is often more of a handicap than the possibility of impotence. Just because someone is in a wheelchair, or has a disability, they should not be denied the same rights to a sex life as anybody else. Carers who can discreetly and sympathetically assist in this without stepping over the professional boundary are invaluable.

Alcohol and narcotics

Too much alcohol has a sedative effect on the body – in fact the body is temporarily poisoned by it, and although women may have sexual intercourse when they are drunk, for men it's more difficult. A little alcohol can greatly enhance an evening, but if you are a heavy drinker, you may begin to realize that whatever you're drinking is disguising another problem, perhaps to do with forming close relationships. Excess alcohol means you often don't get to the point of testing out your sexual prowess even if you do find a partner, and a poisoned body will not function well, even when it comes to having an erection. For narcotics users, impotence is a frequent sequel to heavy use, and loss of desire an even more frequent one. However, you are unlikely to care overmuch about this if you are deeply immersed in this world. Desire and potency may return if the drugs are given up, but sometimes the damage to the body and the mind is too great. There are 'recreational' drugs around said to enhance sexual experience. Cannabis can slow down responses, cocaine and amyl nitrate reportedly produce an intense sensation, but none of these are likely to be helpful to the man with impotence, who needs his body to be in good shape. A person who always needs cannabis, cocaine, amyl nitrate or amphetamines in order to have good sex might benefit from looking at what is really missing in their life. Some diverting activities involving drugs are just this – a way of taking the attention away from the real problem.

Billy and Dawn were a couple who used amphetamine and alcohol at weekends to excess, in order to have exciting sex and to forget about Dawn's dying father whom she cared for during the week. Billy was an alcoholic who had lost his wife and children through a messy divorce caused largely through his drinking. He had modified his drinking a little since then, but experienced episodes of impotence with Dawn. Dawn opted to have counselling on her own and was able to look afresh at her life and the burdens she was carrying. She made a decision to give up using speed and did so, and shortly after that she reported that Billy was making contact with his ex-wife and their children. Dawn realized that the relationship was at an end for the time being. Both had supplied a distraction for the other for as long as it lasted.

Peyronie's Disease

If a man notices a small lump on the side of his penis, which prevents the skin from stretching as it should, so that his penis becomes slightly bent, it's likely he has Peyronie's Disease. This patch of plaque is harmless and only becomes a problem if his penis erects at such an angle that he cannot insert it comfortably into his partner. If you have a bent penis, you should have it checked out by your doctor, who will be able to advise you about treatment if it is needed. By itself it does not usually prevent an erection from occurring, but it may inhibit the man psychologically.

3

What's on offer? Some helpful aids

Let's consider some of the gizmos, gadgets and self-administered drugs that are around at this present time. Because there is a huge amount of money to be made by pharmaceutical companies and prosthetics manufacturers, the market is constantly changing to accommodate the latest drugs and devices. We will look at the basic categories of help, and how they work.

The wonder drug being promoted a few years ago was papaverine, an opiate derivative, which could be injected by the man into his penis and which would dilate the blood vessels of the penis, causing an erection. It proved reliable in doing this for the majority of men without major tissue damage. One drawback was that some men did not lose their erection even after ejaculation, which was dangerous, as over-extended and engorged blood vessels can be damaged by a prolonged erection and need medical intervention to resolve. This effect was not common. Repeated injections can, of cause, create scar tissue after a time and further damage the organ. The thought of an injection into that part of the body as a prelude to love-making is not attractive to many men or their partners. However, it has been reported that for men who had lost their confidence in their ability to maintain an erection, but where there was no physical cause, one or two injections created confidence and no further assistance was necessary. Before the advent of papaverine and Viagra, a substance called catherides or 'Spanish fly' was known to cause sexual excitement, sometimes priapism (a prolonged and painful erection), but regulating the dose was almost impossible. Clearly man's search for an answer to this vexing condition is an ancient one.

Diet is certainly worth a further look, as anyone under stress may not be maintaining their body very well, and vitamins and minerals necessary for healthy function can be missing from our over-refined or unbalanced foodstuffs. Men tend to dismiss this as not having any bearing on their state of health or sexual prowess, but diet is important in maintaining good health. There are several preparations on the market that consist of combinations of herbal drugs and/or vitamins. Some of these preparations have a known effectiveness on certain conditions, such as the properties of tomato and saw palmetto in preventing and relieving prostate problems, or Vitamin E in maintaining good circulation, all of which may have an effect upon the health of the sexual organs. Yohimbine, a herbal drug used in West Africa, has also been reported to increase libido and is a common, though often optional, ingredient of the combination drugs described above. It is unlicensed in the UK, as it can interfere with the effects of other medication. No multi-vitamin or herbal preparation can take the place of a good diet, however, though it may supplement it.

Infertile couples have certainly been helped to improve their chances of conception by changes in their diet and lifestyle. However, most younger men who have a good varied diet, including plenty of fresh fruit and vegetables, and who look after themselves in other ways, are unlikely to benefit greatly from these preparations, although there are tests available from good herbalists and allergy clinics that can pinpoint deficiencies in a person's chemical and mineral balance. It can be dangerous to self-medicate, and you need to be very sure of the credentials and professional standing of any individuals promoting these products, as well as asking your doctor's advice.

Viagra (sildenafil) and other oral medication

Following the advent of papaverine, which is still used in combination with other drugs, Viagra and apomorphine, known under the brand name of Uprima, have proved more popular as a self-administered treatment, as they depend on tablets, not injections, and are reported to work in addition for women who are normally unable to become sexually aroused. Uprima is taken in the form of tablets dissolved under the tongue and starts to take effect after 20 minutes, while Viagra takes a little longer, as the tablets are swallowed and have to be digested. New on the market is Cialis, marketed in France as 'Le Weekend' pill; this has an added advantage of extended effectiveness, over 24 hours, as opposed to Viagra which takes effect in under an hour, removing some of the spontaneity of love-making, which has to be planned and timed to coincide with the effects of the tablet.

Viagra and Uprima (which is still under trial in this country) are not suitable for everyone, however, though if suitable they can be obtained without too much difficulty from clinics and your GP. This treatment is not generally free, except to a few categories of patients with chronic conditions known to cause impotence or where deep distress can be proven. Consequently, it is usually prescribed under a private prescription, and it costs around £20 a time. Viagra should never be taken without medical supervision, as for people with certain medical conditions, such as angina, it can be very dangerous. There are also sometimes unpleasant side-effects, which may include headaches, dizziness or nausea. Both Viagra and Uprima depend on sufficient sexual stimulation to work effectively. Viagra has had remarkable success since it was developed originally as a drug to treat heart disease, and most impotent men can be treated with it. It is important to state that any treatment for impotence is not just a case of taking a tablet, or injecting yourself; there are other considerations too.

Self-injection therapy

A small amount of this drug, usually alprostadil, known under the trade names of Caverject and Edex, is injected into the base of the penis. This treatment is effective even where Viagra has been tried without success. Occasionally it may be mixed with papaverine. Self-injections are said to be no more painful than pinching an ear lobe, but for men with needle phobia the idea of self-injection is frightening in the extreme.

An erection that lasts too long is a rare complication; a man who has an erection lasting longer than three hours should seek urgent medical help. Despite the reservations about injections, to couples for whom Viagra does not work this treatment offers a real alternative which is as close to full unassisted sexual intercourse as it's possible to get. It does have to be prescribed by your doctor or other medical specialist, and full instructions given in its use.

Transurethral therapy

A tiny pellet of alprostadil, known under the brand name Muse, is placed in the urethra with a special applicator. This can create a slight burning sensation, or irritation, both in the man and in his partner, but approximately half the men using it claim to achieve successful intercourse. The drug is absorbed into the bloodstream directly from the urethra. It is not appropriate for men with damage to the blood vessels of the penis.

Vacuum devices

These devices, which vary slightly in their effectiveness and manufacture, work on the principle of drawing blood into the penis by suction, creating a vacuum, and trapping the blood inside the penis by means of a constricting ring around the base. The suction device is then removed. Because an erection is caused by blood being pumped into the penis, this device mimics the natural process. The constricting ring has to be removed after a while to allow the blood to drain away, which can limit the amount of time in which the erection is maintained. Failure to remove the ring would cause damage to the blood vessels, which may already be damaged as a result of illness. What is good about the device is that the penis looks normal when erect, albeit not quite as firm as before, and only the ring around the base is visible. Ejaculation and sensitivity can be slightly affected.

Another similar device is like a condom, from which the air is removed by means of a small pump, the vacuum created being filled with blood being drawn into the penis through the corpora cavernosa, the spongy expanding vessels either side of the penis. This has the advantage that if the erection begins to diminish slightly, the pump can be used briefly to renew it. No one who has normally functioning blood vessels and nerve endings needs to use such a device, but for men who have had bowel surgery, for example, when there is often nerve damage preventing arousal, or for men with cardio-vascular disease, these are useful gadgets worth considering. There are virtually no side-effects and they are safe to use, if used properly; visually they are acceptable.

Implants

There are a number of prosthetic rod implants available which can be surgically implanted into the main blood vessels of the penis. These devices are semi rigid; that is, they can be manually raised or lowered, and when raised the penis is rigid enough for penetration. What is lost is the difference in size and length in a healthy penis that occurs on arousal. Ejaculation may or may not happen, but sexual intercourse is possible. Surgery of this type involves the destruction of the cell walls, which would normally contain the blood, in order to accommodate the rod. Implants are usually only offered as a last resort.

There are also inflatable implants, which are operated by squeezing a small pump situated in the scrotum. This releases fluid that is pumped into two cylinders implanted in the penis, duplicating the blood flow that would occur in a healthy penis. All of this mechanism is internal.

For both types of implants, there are things that can go wrong, though these days this is less common. Rods can snap or break through the wall of the penis and protrude, infections can develop, and sensation can be lost by the damage to nerve endings during the implantation surgery. Psychosexual therapists are sometimes called upon to deal with the distress of these patients when things have gone wrong, when perhaps a better option for them would have been some less invasive and drastic solution. Damage is generally irreversible. These prosthetic devices are also extremely costly, but for some men who want an instant erection they provide a solution.

4

Psychological factors

When we look at impotence that has suddenly occurred, and where there is no illness present, we find that there are a number of triggers that are frequently responsible for loss of desire and impotence. We will look at these and evaluate their outcomes and effects upon the couples concerned. In this chapter I have classed clinical depression as a psychological problem, though it is often classified as a physical one.

Confidence

Regarding confidence, and the loss of it (such a key element in erectile difficulty), it seems that a cycle of repeated failure can become self-fulfilling and hard to escape from. We will consider this first, as whatever the trigger for the initial episode, the blow to self-confidence puts doubt in the mind and allows uncertainty and fear to take hold. Restoring self-confidence is the key to any successful treatment of impotence.

The cycle of hope, attempt, failure and disappointment

Charles, a company manager in his forties, faced a complaint about his handling of a situation at work. Ashamed to tell his wife, Pam, he arranged a night out for Pam's birthday and both set out to enjoy the evening. During the evening, they bumped into someone they knew who asked about the work situation. Pam was angry that Charles hadn't told her, and although they patched things up there was still anger between them when they went to bed. Possibly against his better judgement, Charles tried to make love to Pam, who was lukewarm at first, then became enthusiastic. At this point Charles lost his erection, and Pam, still smarting from previous events, was a little sarcastic. They went to sleep without having really resolved anything. Things dragged on at work and the complaint went up to a higher level. Charles felt threatened on all sides, even though he did not believe there was any foundation to the complaint. The next time they attempted to make love, both were on edge and slightly fearful that it would happen again. It did, and Charles became very depressed, thinking that his career and his marriage would now surely end. This self-defeating attitude exasperated Pam, who in many ways was a more robust character. Further attempts reinforced the failure until they finally gave up trying. Pam by this time was trying to be understanding, but underneath was still quite angry with him. The complaint at work was then resolved and he was exonerated. The fear of sexual failure, however, was by then so reinforced by repeated failed attempts that, despite his confidence at work being partly restored, it was a long time before his sexual potency returned.

Depression

Although medication can often alleviate the symptoms of depression somewhat, and the impotence, if present, may disappear, it might be helpful here to look at depression for which the man does not seek or accept help from his GP. I believe that depression is a major cause or consequence of impotence. Usually it is associated with loss, disappointment or some fundamental realization about the realities of life and death. This may sound morbid, but we can usually fend off the knowledge of our own mortality when we are young. Then something changes. Life seems pointless and futile, the future seems bleak and dread becomes a constant companion. No wonder sex suffers. Losing a job, a parent, a child, a part of your life, involves change and letting go. Depression is often a sequel. Losing economic status and professional status can drain the sexual confidence too. As we saw at the start of this book, there are questions to be asked. Counselling is usually helpful, if it can be accepted. Men unsure about counselling or therapy might consider arranging a limited number of sessions with a suitable therapist to see how they feel about it. After three sessions you should know if it's going to be valuable.

Childbirth and associated gynaecological problems

Childbirth is messy, often painful, and associated with emotional trauma. Females forget the pain, indignity and exhaustion of labour quickly; after all, they have a brand new baby as a reward. For the mother giving birth and lying flat on her back, it is difficult to see what's going on at the business end even if she is propped up, as her belly is in the way. All the mother's energy goes into surviving this experience and pushing the newborn out into the world alive and healthy. Not so for the father. Nurses and midwives often sensibly advise the father to stay at the head end, as the possibility of him fainting while watching the process from the other end is very real. Even so, many men who have been at the births of their babies have mixed feelings about the experience. A particularly difficult birth, involving pain for the mother and a protracted delivery, can turn many men off sex, not to mention their wives. The fear of rupturing stitches or causing damage is a great inhibitor for couples, and this fear extends into pregnancy too, as the presence of a stranger inside the body of his wife may make intercourse impossible for a man.

Most couples overcome these difficulties by uniting in the care of their baby, and let things settle down so that they feel ready to have sex again when their bodies and minds are comfortable with the idea.

For men, and there are some, who have been deeply shocked by the whole experience of childbirth, the fear of making their partner pregnant again is always present, despite contraception. This, too, can switch off desire very effectively.

Other gynaecological problems women experience can turn men off sex, even if the woman is willing and able. I marvel at the endurance of the woman with endometriosis who, despite frequent bleeds, made love often with her husband and kept a set of old towels to hand to put under her bottom to catch any leakages. Her husband, a very loving man, understood that there wasn't a lot she could do about the condition and, provided the experience was pleasurable and not painful for them both, was happy to proceed. For the husband who cannot bring himself to make love to his partner following her hysterectomy or other operation, this is a real hurdle to overcome. No wonder many couples call it a day at that point and pay the emotional cost rather than attempt a sexual life together.

This is where the district nurse or doctor can make a real difference by asking discreetly about the sexual functioning of the couple and not making assumptions. It's usually a huge relief to have the opportunity to discuss this.

Assault and rape

It is quite common for the partners of women who have been raped to become impotent for a while. Fathers of girls who have been raped may also suffer in this way. It is also not uncommon for partners faced with a disclosure by their partner of sexual abuse, to avoid sex. They may, after all, be replicating behaviour their partner found deeply repugnant or traumatizing. While rape victims are often offered help in the form of supportive counselling, their partners often suffer acutely on their own, being unable to help, and feeling themselves to be identified with the aggressor by virtue of being male. The feelings of powerlessness and guilt at what they may see as their failure to protect their partner are very strong in most male partners of rape victims. One of the most powerful torture tools employed by sadistic regimes is to rape the wife or lover of the man you are holding prisoner, without him being able to do anything to prevent it. This is no less true in individual cases of rape.

Women who have been sexually abused as children may or may not let their partner know what happened to them. If a disclosure is made, it may well be at a time of heightened emotional significance for the woman, such as after the death of the abuser, and it will have an impact on their partner and their relationship. Things may now make sense that never did before. Why did she always insist on making love in the morning and never at night? Why did she so dislike him approaching her from behind? Why did she always sleep with her light on? Suddenly the answers are clear.

Maybe he feels he may have been unwittingly molesting her, and if he's known the abuser as one of her family members he now has to rethink that relationship and deal with his own rage and fury at what has happened. Impotence is often a sequel, until the relationship has been renegotiated. Because flashbacks are common and cause panic and anxiety, both parties need reassurance and permission to stop what they're doing at any time during love-making in order to contain the feelings that will arise. Learning to ride through this fear safely, with the partner of their choice supporting them, is for many women the most final way of claiming back what the abuse robbed them of – the right to enjoy their own sexuality without fear, with their partner.

Fertility problems

Couples who have a fertility problem, where IVF is offered, have to make love on demand, attending to temperature, monthly cycle and their general health in a way which makes many relationships hard to sustain as exciting sexual encounters. The whole thing can seem like a chore, and it's not unknown for men to go off sex, though they may masturbate as they did before. The pressure to perform extends to the pressure to conceive as well. If this is the case with you, talk to the clinic about it, and arrange, if it's possible, to take some time off from the programme to enjoy a normal relationship.

Geoff became impotent when, after years of trying to conceive with his wife, he reluctantly went for a sperm count and found that his count was low and his sperm unviable. The news that he was extremely unlikely to father a child made his wife very angry, as she felt he had wasted a lot of her time by not having the test before, even though she too had problems with her fallopian tubes. The bitterness and disappointment led to a rift in their marriage and to his impotence. As he said, what was the point of intercourse when it didn't result in what they both longed for? By this he really meant his wife and his desire to please her. The relationship broke up, and he then tested out his sexual equipment with another partner and found himself able to function. Children in this relationship were not an issue, but his marriage could not contain the disappointment of childlessness. Knowing his impotence was specific to his marriage helped him to make a more stable and permanent commitment once he had got over his loss and disappointment in respect of his marriage.

Fear of disease

Eric, usually a cautious man and happily married, travelled abroad with his work. Once, on a visit to Thailand, he became drawn in by the sexual freedom on display all around him and enjoyed by the other members of his party. He had always been seen as unadventurous but dependable by his colleagues. This time he allowed himself to become sexually involved with a local woman following a massage, and had been very ashamed the next day. He could have lived with the shame, but what grew inside him and began to gnaw away at him was the fact that he might be infected with AIDS. He confided in a friend and was not offered much consolation. His fear grew. He was unable to make love to his wife on his return and finally went to his doctor, at his wife's insistence, who told him what a test for HIV would entail. He went for the test after much internal dialogue and was clear, but for a while was still impotent. It seemed that he needed to punish himself for what he had done. The thought that the test might not be correct also nagged at him. Finally he permitted himself to believe he was well and began to take the view that he had had a lucky escape. He never did tell his wife, who probably guessed something had happened but decided not to pursue him about it.

Fear is a huge inhibitor in all things sexual. HIV and other sexually transmitted diseases that may not be fatal but will be uncomfortable and difficult to treat, such as herpes, are still on the increase, and if you are worried that you may have caught something, or had unprotected sex, you really should visit a clinic attached to a Department of Genital and Urinary Medicine, usually referred to as a GUM clinic, and talk to someone in the know. Knowing what you're dealing with, even if it's the worst you can imagine, may be better than a lifetime of wondering and fear, not to mention infecting others.

Traumatic sexual injury

It is possible, by too vigorous sexual activity, to break the blood vessels in the penis. This is extremely painful and needs urgent medical treatment. Any extreme pain in the genital region is likely to make the owner of the gonads in question extremely cautious about intercourse. A number of young males I have come across have been inhibited for years in their sexual lives by one very painful episode. Fear, and especially fear of pain, conditions the body in an adverse way. Confidence has to be built up again slowly, with an understanding partner. A sex therapist can be most helpful here, in designing a programme to recondition the sexual responses and eliminate the fear.

Male abuse by females

Although not as common as abuse by males, abuse by females does occur. It is underreported, in my view, because the myth still exists that if a young boy is excited by a woman, it must be a good thing. Lucky him, they might say, hearing that a 15-year-old schoolboy has slept with the school nurse. However, it is still sexual abuse and an abuse of power and professional trust. The boy who is aroused and excited by female babysitters, his sister's friends, teachers or others older than himself, when this excitement is taken advantage of and acted upon, is left with a complicated and troubling set of responses to females, and if a female partner in later life unwittingly replicates this situation, the man may find the interaction so troubling that he becomes impotent. Men who have experienced seductive mothers, or who have been humiliated sexually by mothers or sisters, more frequently experience delayed ejaculation with their partners. They become erect but unable to ejaculate inside their partner. If this leads to difficulty between them, possibly because she wants to become pregnant or doesn't understand his problem, he may lose his erections altogether. Desire becomes a frightening and unhappy state, and the taboos, fears and inhibitions sometimes become too strong to manage. Some of the most unhappy and troubled young men I have met have been the victims of female abuse of one sort or another, but because of the myths around male sexuality and the false supposition that for males any sex is to be welcomed and enjoyed, even if it actually makes you feel sick inside, it is difficult for males to come forward for help in untangling this and ridding themselves of the effects of their abuse. Men are not supposed to feel frightened, ashamed or vulnerable in our culture, though thankfully this is beginning to change.

Male abuse by males

Males who have been abused early in their lives by men are coming forward more frequently now, and society has to take note of their distress. What they experience may or may not affect their performance in sexual relationships with women, though it always affects their lives adversely in other ways. If you feel that your mother should have protected you and/or noticed something was wrong, you may carry this anger with you into your marriage and become unable to give yourself fully to your partner. Mostly, males who are predominantly heterosexual are not affected in their sexual performance with a female partner by past abuse from a male, but emotionally they may well be deeply affected. Certainly there is often a crisis of sexual orientation, especially if the abuse occurred at adolescence, when they had strong same-sex relationships and experienced a certain amount of sexual excitement in them, which is normal for that age. Abuse subverts the normal development of sexual orientation and identity, and unwilling sexual arousal, which often happens in abusive situations as a normal bodily response, leads to great confusion in young males. The doubt about whether he is really as male as he should be, if he has experienced past arousal by males, makes sexual relationships with women tricky. Sometimes there is a need to prove one's heterosexuality many times, with many different partners, as a way of re-patterning the sexual arousal triggers, and the penis may not always agree with this attitude and refuse eventually to obey.

There is a different type of male abuse that affects a man, and that is the physical or sexual abuse of his mother by the dominant male in the household. The fear, excitement and horror of hearing or witnessing, as a child, your mother being forced to endure sexual acts as part of a violent relationship, will have an effect in conditioning your sexual arousal patterns in a way that will probably be most uncomfortable for you. If this has been your experience, and you recognize it has had an effect on you, I urge you to seek a good therapist to work with. You do not need to suffer alone with this, and if you are lucky enough to have found a relationship that is loving, and where your sexual partner is puzzled by your sexual behaviour, your anxiety or your fear, now is the time to seek assistance. Only when we feel safe enough in the present can we go back and re-work the past.

Anger with a partner

John's wife Gayle had an affair with a man John had always admired and who was a family friend. John's anger and distress

33

was such that, despite his wife ending the affair and feeling deeply unhappy about what had happened, he was unable to make love to her. Partly he was deeply blocked by his own anger and sense of betrayal; partly he did not want to put his penis in a place where the other man's penis had been. His wife felt unforgiven and upset, yet was frightened of resuming their sexual relationship. A collusion developed between them to avoid sexual contact, and as time passed his impotence began to trouble him more and more. As they began to heal a little from the wounds they had inflicted on one another, and it seemed as though the sexual side might become viable again, he began to fear it all the more. After all, she had preferred the other man. What if he could not compete? A sex therapist helped them to start again and unravel the left-over pain and anger, doubt and confusion, until they were able to approach their sex life again by degrees and claim it back for themselves. Initially they were instructed not to attempt intercourse, but to concentrate instead on mutual pleasuring and making time and space for one another. As the lack of this previously had led to the affair, restoring it in their marriage was vital. Trust and confidence grew between them and they regained their fondness and need for one another sexually, and became sexual partners once again.

Change in body image and loss of confidence

Because impotence and loss of confidence are so closely bound up together, any change perceived as negative in a man with low self-esteem can lead to a lack of sexual confidence. Baldness, weight gain, disability or the ageing process can sometimes undermine the confidence of the man sexually. If his partner is less than kind and he feels bad about himself, he is less likely to want sex or maintain his erection with his partner. This reinforces the failure and makes matters worse. Some things cannot be changed, only made the best of, but we all change as we grow older and have to adjust continually to the physical changes age brings. If a partner changes greatly in their appearance this may also lead to a diminishing of sexual attraction and even aversion. One man, greatly ashamed to admit how he felt, stated that his wife had gained 4 stone in weight and 'it wasn't what I signed up for'. He still loved her, but was put off by her sudden increase in size. Another man, attracted by larger women, would not have had this problem; sexual attraction and desire are very complex, individual things.

As we have seen, there are many situations and combinations of events that can lead to loss of desire and erection problems. A great many of these are temporary, but may cause great unhappiness while they last.

Same-sex attraction

There are bi-sexual or gay men living in heterosexual relationships for whom the sex act becomes harder and harder to manage with their female partner. The partner may be greatly loved, but the relationship will suffer sexually. Homosexual feelings, denied at first, will be the focus of masturbatory fantasy and can cause intense conflict and depression in the man. As his homosexual feelings become stronger, and same-sex sexual acts occur with more frequency outside the home, it may become impossible to make love to the female partner any more. At a certain point, a decision has to be reached between the two as to whether they continue to live together. Some couples can accommodate this, with the man finding sexual satisfaction outside the marriage while staying with his wife. He may or may not be impotent with a male partner, but he is quite likely to become impotent with his female one. Same-sex couples where one is experiencing impotence are open to the same types of treatment as any other couples. One aspect of this might be to do with the difficulty some men have in finding love and sex in the same place, and the availability of casual sex for gay men, without their committed relationship being threatened.

Strong religious influences

Sexual problems among devoutly religious people are often made more difficult to resolve because of the strongly held beliefs and views of adherents. A man who has been trained in a seminary to switch off or sublimate his sexual feelings may find it difficult to allow them free expression with a partner if he leaves the seminary or the priesthood. Desire is switched off almost before it has been registered. Consequently men from backgrounds where sexual taboos are strong, masturbation is prohibited and sexual intercourse is only allowed within very defined parameters, are likely to experience some problems. Impotence may alternate with premature ejaculation, and retarded ejaculation may become impotence. Desire and arousal may fluctuate widely, depending on the circumstances, and anger, self-blame and guilt add fuel to the fire. Anger with the other party who has tempted them, or created feelings of desire, may make intercourse a desperate, angry, shameful affair. In cultures, including our own, where women are generally expected to be submissive to the will of the man, it may be difficult for the woman to express her feelings openly and an impotent husband could be affected by his wife's unexpressed anger, just as she may be affected by his impotence.

A distorted view of women as either madonnas or whores, temptresses or virgins in some religious societies, makes it difficult for the man to put his penis into this holy receptacle, thereby defiling it, or into this filthy and shameful place, thereby soiling himself.

The prognosis for men from strict religious backgrounds and who are impotent is not good, unless the relationship they have with their partner becomes more realistic and relaxed. Any deeply religious man seeking help from a sex therapist for impotence should check that the therapist respects his religious beliefs and is willing to work with them. This is particularly true for followers of Islam, where there are a number of restrictions on certain activities that may make traditional sex therapy difficult to engage with.

5
Mind or body, or both?

If you, or your partner, are troubled by erection problems or loss of desire for love-making, there is quite a lot of self-assessment you can do. Talking through these questions with your partner or someone trained to assess sexual problems can be very helpful. Absolute honesty is required! If you have a sneaking suspicion that the problem may not be purely physical, look at the assessment anyway, but don't hesitate in getting checked out by the doctor if problems persist; in fact, this is what most men would want to do first.

Questions

1 Think back to the first time you really noticed that it happened. Where were you? What had happened that day? How was it different from other times? What sort of mood were you in? What sort of mood was your partner in?
2 In the weeks and months leading up to this point, what was your work schedule like? How busy were you, and how tired?
3 What was your state of health like in the period before the problem began? If you are athletic or work in a manual job, did you with hindsight exert yourself more than you normally would?
4 Did any major change occur in your life before the onset of this problem? What was it, and how much thinking time did it take up?
5 Do you still masturbate? If so, can you get and maintain an erection without problems? How often does this happen? If you get regular erections when on your own, then the problem is unlikely to be a medical one, though it may be caused by depression.
6 Has anything happened to knock your confidence? (Be truthful!)
7 How much alcohol do you consume? Did the amount increase prior to the onset of the problem?

8 Are you a smoker? If you smoke heavily it is likely that this will affect your ability to maintain an erection. Cut down and see if it makes a difference.

9 How well are you getting along with your partner? Periods of stress and tension with no dialogue between you can be very damaging to the sexual life of any couple.

10 How well are you sleeping? Are you always tired, or sleeping but waking in the night? Has your sleep pattern changed? If the answer is yes and you feel constantly weary, ask yourself if you might be depressed or anxious about something. Again, talking about it helps. Depression is, I believe, a major cause, or maintainer, of impotence. Most thinking people suffer from occasional periods of depression, usually linked to a loss of some sort, or being trapped in a situation they have no control over. It will pass, especially if you make a decision to examine what's going on and make some changes. Loss has to be lived with, but the feelings that surround it may change over time, especially if you can take the stuff clogging up your internal world and externalize it. If talking therapies are not your cup of tea there are other alternatives. Writing or drawing it out can help to unblock the awful depressed feelings, though I have to say that having someone there with you to support you and offer a different perspective is extremely useful. Let your doctor know about it, especially if it interferes with your sleep and you have a dead, grey feeling of dread that stays with you, or you entertain thoughts about harming yourself or feel life is not worth living. This is serious and needs treatment. A very helpful book on this subject is Dorothy Rowe's *Depression: The Way Out of Your Prison*, listed at the end of this book.

11 Does the situation change when you are away from your usual setting? There are couples who only make love during holidays away from home with their partner. Is someone living with you or near you who inhibits your sexual life – a parent or teenage child, for example? How did home become associated with a lack of sex?

12 What experiences are you and your partner carrying with you from previous sexual relationships? Is your performance something you worry about?

13 Are you taking 'recreational drugs'? Heroin is known to affect

libido and sexual function, for example, while amphetamine and cocaine are reported to increase desire and arousal, overriding the body's own normal desires for sex, food, sleep or emotional fulfilment. Even cannabis can interfere with this more than regular users realize. The physical changes brought about by regular drug use throw the body out of gear and disturb natural rhythms; this can be hard to remedy.

14 Lastly, what would change if you did not have this problem?

Answering these questions fully will give you some clues about what it was that was going on in your life that led up to this point. Exhaustion, mental and physical, affects the penis. If the brain says, 'Sleep is what I need, not sex, right now,' and a man tries to override this, his penis may not obey him.

Having read this far and identified a number of reasons for the erectile difficulty, you may be wondering: 'What now? It's all very well identifying the causes, but I'm still stuck with the problem.' Assuming that you have been checked out by the doctor, you may decide to go down one of a number of routes. The larger drug companies will try to entice you down many expensive routes, not all of them orthodox. Be cautious. Your doctor will only prescribe drugs known to be safe for you in the light of his present knowledge. Wonder drugs are seldom anything of the kind, whereas drugs such as Viagra are known to be effective but have their limitations. They have been subjected to extensive medical trials before being offered to patients. Viagra will only enable an erection if there is enough sexual stimulation present. And if part of you is really saying, 'I can't be bothered', stimulation is unlikely to work.

Another, more lengthy but successful route is to ask for a referral to a psychosexual clinic. Local health services operate clinics around the country, staffed by well-trained practitioners, but the service is patchy. Not all practitioners are trained in marital relationships, however, and as this can be a crucial aspect of the problem, it's advisable to check this out with the therapist. Relate offers a service to couples and some individuals, which combines sex therapy with an understanding and knowledge of the dynamics of couple relationships. They are very successful in the work they do. This service is not free, and patients may refer themselves, though GPs often refer their patients to this service and usually have an ongoing professional dialogue with sex therapists in their area. GPs often find the whole area of patient sexuality a difficult one for them to treat, and it isn't given a great deal of attention in medical school, so they are usually happy to refer patients to a sex therapist they know and trust. Sex therapy is discussed more fully in Chapter 8.

A sex therapist should ideally be a member of a professional body called the BASRT, that is the British Association for Sexual and Relationship Therapy. This body updates members regularly on work in the field; it offers regular training events and demands high professional and ethical standards. The contact address for the organization, which is happy to advise you of practitioners working in your area, is at the back of this book. Members may work for agencies such as Relate or London Marriage Guidance, or in the Health Service, in private practice, or both. For more information about the work of a Health Service psychosexual clinic, you may want to look at the website of the Porterbrook Clinic in Sheffield as an example. The address is at the back of this book.

Low testosterone levels

In desperation, some men take to trawling the Internet to see what other solutions might be on offer, besides drugs, prosthetic devices and sex therapy.

One answer seized upon by some is the condition known as 'the male menopause'. Whether this is the same as a mid-life crisis is not clear, but if you consider the fact that work stress has reached huge proportions now, and in mid-life many difficult events coincide – parents die, children leave home but still need financial assistance, teenagers put a strain on the marriage – and add to this redundancy, illness or divorce, all at a time when the body is beginning to be depleted, it's easy to see the sense of this reasoning. But the answer to the male menopause or mid-life crisis is not in a pill, unless you're ill, but in changing your lifestyle, taking better care of yourself and allowing yourself a chance to recover from what life has thrown at you. What is usually offered instead is a testosterone boost, under a variety of brand names, which may make you feel great for a short while but, because the body develops a dependency, cannot continue indefinitely.

Many men with slightly lowered levels of testosterone are not impotent – far from it – so it isn't by any means always a sequel. Stress, fatigue, depression and poor self-care are far more likely to be responsible for impotence, and this does need you to do something about it.

Physical and mental illness

If you are impotent because of a physical illness (excluding clinical depression), it's likely you'll be offered some advice, counselling and/or hands-on medical treatment. If you are clinically depressed and impotent, the chances are that you may not care that much, except for the effect on your partner. You may be offered medication, psychotherapy or counselling as part of your treatment. Until you recover from the depression, you are unlikely to recover from the impotence. If you have a mental illness, such as schizophrenia or bi-polar disorder, you may well be in a stable and satisfactory sexual relationship, providing your illness is well managed, but major tranquillizers *can* cause erection problems and loss of libido, though the effects of lithium-based drugs on sexual behaviour do not seem to be significant. There are alternative medications on the market for people who have experienced psychotic breakdowns, and some of the newer drugs are free from the side-effects experienced with traditional medication. Doctors are not mind-readers; they cannot know about the effects of the illness and medication on your relationship unless they are told. If you can't talk to your doctor about this, ask to be referred to someone you *can* talk to. If you have a community psychiatric nurse who visits you, you could start by asking them, or by phoning a helpline.

Sex therapy can be very helpful in giving you and your partner a place to talk about what you want from a sex life and how to get it, given any restrictions you may now face. A man who has had a heart attack may be scared of any sexual exertion. His partner may be even more afraid that sexual activity will precipitate another attack. A person who has an epileptic seizure during sexual activity, or experiences any other abnormal state, may scare their partner more than themselves. The humiliation and embarrassment may, however, be equally significant in the long run.

Performance anxiety

Performance anxiety is one of the most important aspects of erectile dysfunction where there is no organic cause. The aim of a sex therapist would be to assist you both to overcome this anxiety and learn new ways of relaxing, self-calming and unhurried love-making. If we were brought up in homes that expected us to do nothing less than our best in everything, and expected instant results, our own performance standards may be very high. We can help ourselves here, by learning relaxation techniques and rethinking some of our attitudes. Partners too can often make good use of these techniques, and this is part and parcel of what the sex therapist can offer, though there are other places where this can be explored, through stress management or other courses.

Ageing

Occasional erectile dysfunction is more likely to happen the older you get. Just as we can no longer expect to run as fast as we did in our twenties, it's unreasonable to expect that a penis will maintain Olympic standards all the time when you are older. It's just life, and it only becomes a problem if it gets in the way of your relationship. The conditions for good sex may not be there. A great deal depends on the man's state of health and fitness. There are, anyway, some positive benefits from being older. An older man is unlikely to experience premature ejaculation. His erection may well last longer, and his patience and awareness of his own and his partner's needs will be a real bonus. He may also have had the important realization that there's no rush. So what if he's lost his erection? He'll have another. Relax.

Unfortunately, in our youth- and celebrity-obsessed media, the notion of older people enjoying good sex is not well presented. However, the truth is that a couple who have enjoyed their sexual relationship all the way through their marriage are likely, health permitting, to carry on enjoying it well into old age. There is a security and trust with a partner with whom you have enjoyed a long-term relationship. Arousal and excitement are conditioned into the relationship, which is very healthy. If a partner dies, the loss of this in a partner with whom there was a satisfying sexual relationship is hard for others to appreciate if the couple are elderly. The general loss will be understood, but as to the sexual loss, it isn't 'nice' to talk about it, but it's still a very significant part of their bereavement. Loyalty to the deceased partner can prevent the man making another sexual relationship. Missing a sexual partner may also lead to inappropriate sexual advances towards people who do not welcome it.

Older people can and do fall in love, enjoy their sexual lives, and begin new ones with different partners if the opportunity presents itself. I'm not suggesting that this needs to be put under the noses of younger people, only acknowledged. It seems to me that too many assumptions are made about older people, as they are about the disabled, and that each individual is exactly that – an individual.

With this in mind, it really does make sense for couples requesting help with erectile dysfunction (or any other sexual dysfunction) to have the best possible assessment with a skilled practitioner. Several therapists report that men sometimes come to the clinic wanting individual help, usually a quick fix. These men want to leave their partners out of the equation. If Viagra is tried and the man does not become aroused, as he may not, what then? Therapy with these men is usually unsuccessful, as they fear engaging in a joint dialogue with their wife or partner about what is very much a joint activity.

Information

Sometimes women are unaware of what turns their man on; they may be afraid to touch his penis or handle him in a way that excites him. He may be equally unaware how to arouse her. Quite often there is a lot of interesting work to do to fill in the gaps for the couple about these issues. There's no shame in this, for as someone once said to me: 'Sex is the only thing a man is expected to know how to do without anyone ever actually showing him how.' Maybe this statement isn't as true as it was, given the number of self-help sex videos around, but an average couple who do not want to seek out very explicit material, designed to excite rather than instruct, are left with material that leaves a lot to be desired in terms of clarity. With a sex therapist, there is time to learn and ask questions without a pornographic content or embarrassment. It's very different from the sex education most of us had at school – something I recall being all about rabbits, sperm and ovum and nothing at all about the erect penises, the clitoris or masturbation, which, being female, was what I wanted to know about.

Anger

If there is left-over anger in the relationship, this too will need defusing if it gets in the way of good sex. A person does not want to have sex with someone they dislike or about whom they have a negative opinion. If you have a row and clear the air, then there's no better way of making up, but when something has festered on for a long time and never been dealt with, sex often becomes a no-go area. Sex can be withheld as a punishment or given as a reward, rather than experienced as a mutually rewarding activity. An exasperated man once commented to me that requesting sex with his wife was like demanding to borrow the crown jewels. This preciousness and grudging attitude, beset by terms and conditions, spelled the death of the marriage eventually.

A spouse who dislikes sex or has another person in her life she is paying more attention to, whether it's their child, her boss, her father or a lover, will find her partner suffering from lack of interest, or becoming angry as a result of deprivation. Most men can cope with their wife giving all her attention to their newborn, but when the 15-year-old son takes the place of the father, and becomes her soul mate, companion and defender, the marriage is in real trouble and the chances are that sex will have ceased quite a while before, often at the instigation of the man. Although this isn't strictly speaking erectile dysfunction, there is a fine line between lack of desire and impotence.

6

The role of relationships in erectile dysfunction

Confidence is so important in relationships where erectile dysfunction has occurred that we need to look more closely at the power and control issues in the relationship as a whole to see how it may affect the sexual functioning.

Trevor, always a timid man, had married Sonia when they were both young. Sonia was forceful and ambitious and continued to get promotion at work. She began to earn far more than Trevor, who was a carpet fitter for a local firm and more or less contented to stay where he was. As her life became busier and busier, she found it hard to relax at home and began to demean Trevor in front of her friends. He hated this, but said nothing. He tried to help her more at home, but could never get it right. Both became increasingly unhappy. Then his firm put him on a three-day week and his self-confidence really began to suffer.

He began to experience episodes of impotence on the rare occasions they attempted intercourse. They had hoped to start a family, and the infrequency and unsatisfactory nature of their love-making meant that this had become another disappointment and cause of lack of confidence between them. Trevor took all the blame, while Sonia gave out all the anger and disappointment. Finally Trevor went to his doctor, who was shrewd enough to realize that this was a problem between Trevor and his wife, and referred them for counselling. Trevor's wife refused to attend, saying it was his problem, but Trevor found that the opportunity to discuss his fears in private gave him the confidence to approach Sonia in a different way, and he began to be more assertive. Sonia, thoroughly angry by now and upset that he was talking about her to a stranger, told him to leave. His confidence knocked again, Trevor still persevered with his more confident assertive style and began another relationship after an interval. He was not impotent in this relationship, as the woman he was involved with was kind and affirming. Sonia, seeing him positive and happier than he had been with her, wanted him back, but he decided not to take the risk of it happening again.

A son taking his father's place

Betty and Jack, a couple in their sixties, had not been on friendly terms for years, living in a cat and dog marriage which, although bad, they couldn't end. Their son Jason, 36, came back to live with them after his marriage failed. He and his mother became constant companions, and Jason became a surrogate husband. Jack got pushed to the side more and more but dared not tackle his son directly. When Jason returned to the family home their sex life, which had until then provided them with a way of making up, stopped. Only when Jason went on holiday were they free enough to have a truce. They tried to resume their sex life, but Jack found himself unable to get an erection. He felt under pressure and there was too much lost ground to make up. Betty saw this as further evidence of his not caring for her and the couple became even more unhappy.

Finally Jack moved out of the bedroom and into the box room. Jason, feeling himself caught up in a difficult situation with his parents, began to think about moving out and finally did so. Jack's erections did not return, however, but Betty preferred it that way, blaming him for the loss of their son. Sadly, they remained stuck like this, as so many couples choose to do.

A younger partner

Fred, 62, divorced his wife of 30 years to set up home with an employee, Susie, 27, who was the same age as his daughter. His ex-wife and children refused all contact with him. Susie was attractive and sex was fine.

Then one day, when her friends had been round to visit, he overheard a comment about the difference in their ages. Later, he looked at himself in the mirror and saw himself as he truly was – paunch, bags under the eyes, greying hair – and experienced a huge and sudden loss of confidence. Susie began to be irritated by his old-fashioned approach to things, the way he wouldn't make love with the light on, his dislike of her friends, the way he sometimes reminded her of her father. He began to experience episodes of impotence and became quite desperate. If he couldn't keep Susie, who did he have left? No one. He became depressed and drank heavily. The impotence increased. Finally he went to his doctor, who suggested they try Viagra. Although Susie loved him, she had to force herself to respond to him sexually, and eventually they ceased trying. The Viagra worked some of the time, but not enough for Fred to feel really confident again. Fred was quite wealthy, and was never sure if this was the reason Susie stayed with him, despite his impotence.

It's so much simpler for the man to say, 'It's my problem and I'll go and get a tablet from the doctor to cure it,' than it is to say, 'There are things going on here that I don't understand, and I need to spend time, energy and probably money in discovering what these are and what to do about it.' Marriages are tricky beasts: nudge them one way and they'll fall over, nudge them another and they'll explode, or start to blossom, or fall into a hole never to be seen again. A good therapist will hold things steady, enabling you both to have a good look at what's going on and make a detailed assessment of the difficulty, before attempting to treat it.

Dominant female partners

A woman who is quite forceful or demanding in attitude and style, and who shows little vulnerability, may make a quieter, more laid-back partner feel thoroughly inadequate. There are some relationships where this go-getting aspect of the female is a major part of the attraction, but the sexual relationship is likely to be problematic unless she is able to maintain his confidence in his sexual ability. It may be that sex is the only area of the marriage where the man feels adequate and in control. If this fails, the relationship will hit major problems. It's easy to feel indignation and anger with the wife who frequently undermines the confidence of her partner (and it happens the other way round as well, of course), but unless the therapist can win the female partner over and understand her feelings too, things are unlikely to mend. Many dominant females long for a more equal relationship and secretly want their husbands to stand up to them, sexually as well as verbally. Dominant women have a great deal to offer in a relationship, but only when their partner is able to check them from time to time, and assert himself. The dominant female partner is often quite insecure herself, though if she is never able to show this the balance in the marriage will become so weighted on one side that unless some evening up occurs, both will be unhappy. We learn a great deal from our parents as role models in this respect, and if Dad was passive and anxious to please and Mum was demanding and critical, and we never saw Dad standing up for himself, it's hard to know how to manage this when we have no example to go from.

Robina was a strong-looking, slightly masculine woman of 45. She was married to Alan, 52, and they had boys of 9 and 11. Alan had been in the Merchant Navy when they met and had seen his share of the world, including bars and brothels. Alan looked older than he was, and had taken early retirement when his firm closed down. He was now not working. He let Robina do the talking for them both. Robina was not happy in her marriage. She found Alan to be useless around the house, and although he cooked and cleaned while she worked, she felt she had to follow him round to make sure he did things properly. She and the boys had taken on work at home to help their financial situation, and he did not contribute to this very much. Robina was the more forceful character and despised her husband, but he secretly enjoyed being dominated by her and made no efforts to stand up to her, or to find work. They had not slept together for five years, and Alan had moved into the bedroom of one of their sons. Robina now had a female companion she went out with and with whom she was closer than she was with Alan. Alan was able to get erections on his own with no problem, and the thought of having sex with Robina excited him a great deal, but when it came to the point he backed away, preferring, it seemed, to maintain the slightly sado-masochistic role he had chosen for himself. Robina's relationship with her female friend was intense, but not sexual, and she wanted Alan to rescue her from her own homosexual feelings by meeting her sexual needs. Her demanding and angry attitude towards him ensured that this never happened, and so they were caught in a fixed cycle of unfulfilled sexual yearning, fear and ambivalence. It turned out that both were really asking for permission to stay as they were, as change would have upset the status quo too much. Alan did at least move out of his son's room and into the spare room, and both were concerned about the effect their relationship was having on their boys.

Alan had powerful masturbatory fantasies about what he saw as the dominatrix aspect of his wife, but he couldn't test them out in reality. As being humiliated secretly excited him, and being in control suited her on some level, there was no real incentive to change. Strictly speaking, Alan was not impotent; neither was he complaining of impotence. Robina, however, had him caught in a double bind, aggressively complaining about his shortcomings on one hand, while stating that she wanted him to become a proper husband to her sexually. Yet everything she did or said gave the opposite impression. Alan, it seemed, quite enjoyed the power of withholding sex from her.

Past influences

Sometimes the past intrudes on present relationships. A man whose previous partner has died may experience intense feelings of disloyalty with a new partner as he attempts penetration, especially if he has been faithful to his wife and has had few previous sexual partners. This can cause erection difficulty, until the man is able to give himself permission to move on and take his time with his new partner.

Previous partners leave their memories behind, which may invade the bedroom in a new relationship in a way that brings distress to both partners. He will not be able to talk about this to his new partner, or about how his ex-partner disliked him doing this but insisted he do that, or how humiliated he felt when she found someone else, or how guilty he felt when he did. Once the relationship is strong enough and contains enough trust, it may be possible to talk about it. There's a great deal they will not be able to share initially, because the ghost of the past will need to be banished, not welcomed into this new relationship, and sexual jealousy is so easy to trigger that discussion of past sexual experiences is likely to lead to difficult confrontations.

Comparisons are odious, as they say, and nowhere is this more true than in the area of sexual experience. This is what makes recovery from an affair so difficult in a marriage that is being mended. The wife will feel she is being compared to the other woman and may want to know every detail of what they did together. Generally this is unhelpful and only feeds the flames of curiosity and jealousy. If the man cannot get an erection with his wife, she may think it's because he's comparing her unfavourably with his lover. This may not be true, but the fear it will give rise to in him may well make him impotent. If she was the one who had an affair, he may feel in competition with the other man. She may also want to punish her husband for the feelings of guilt she has. If the husband was already feeling a lack of confidence (and maybe that's why she left him) this will be increased by her anger and resentment. When there has been sexual infidelity, it is very common for the sexual life of the couple to see-saw between intense sexual acting out and no sex at all. Again, depression and emotional exhaustion may lead to temporary impotence, which is quite normal.

Roy and Margaret, a couple in their early sixties, had enjoyed a good sex life together since they married. A religious couple, from a fundamentalist church, they frequently went on church-sponsored outings and holidays together. Roy became friendly with another couple and was attracted by the wife, and Margaret became very jealous, although the relationship was platonic. She began to fear that she was not as attractive as the woman Roy was attracted to, and she disliked Roy seeing her undressed in case he was comparing her with this woman, who was younger than she was. She avoided sexual contact with Roy in many ways, by going to bed early, spending more time with their daughter, and developing mysterious ailments that were off-putting to her husband. The fears about Roy and this other woman began to eat away at her. Roy tried to reassure her. Margaret sought advice from a church elder and was unsatisfied with what she was told. On the one hand it seemed to be a wife's duty to have sex with her husband, but on the other hand she gained the impression that she was not really expected to enjoy it.

Roy talked to her about the meeting and they tried to have intercourse that night. Margaret seemed to be willing, but in the bedroom started talking about the treatment she was having for mouth ulcers, and it effectively put Roy off, so that he lost his erection. This happened several times, with Margaret sabotaging their sex life in a variety of ways, complaining about his approach, her ailments, finding the room too cold or hot, light or dark, or being generally too tetchy to allow him to approach her. His increasing impotence gave her hope that he would cease to find this other woman attractive (and act on it), and she still felt angry with him about it. Roy felt very frustrated by the lack of sex in his marriage and sometimes tormented Margaret with references to the other woman. This increased the anger between them and made sex even more unlikely. Finally Roy saw a counsellor who suggested that as Margaret was getting older, she might see herself as less desirable and the other woman as a threat. He agreed. The counsellor also helped him to question whether he might be partly responsible for Margaret's anger by referring to the other woman at times, knowing it would upset her. He decided, after talking it over, to embark on a process of courtship with her again, not seeking any sexual reward. She was suspicious at first, but was eventually won round by his efforts. She fought a battle within herself when sex became a possibility, but Roy managed to disarm her, going slowly and courting her in the way he had when they were young. It amounted to a seduction, and she felt slightly guilty and yet excited by it when they had finished. Roy had not lost his erection, and she had refrained from sabotaging their sex.

It isn't difficult to put someone off the idea of sex and dampen their arousal. All it takes is a bitter row unresolved, an unfounded criticism or a humiliating remark, among other things, to put a stop to any possible sexual activity. This is true for women as well as men, perhaps more so. If something happens earlier in the day and causes feelings of anger and resentment which are not dealt with, the man will go off the idea of sex before he's even had time to get and lose an erection, while the woman will show by her body language just what she thinks of the situation. If he tries to override his instincts – and her anger – he may get, but then lose, his erection as a consequence.

John, a 32-year-old man with a stammer, became impotent after his aggressive father told his girlfriend he hoped she'd make a man of him. Luckily he'd met the right woman and eventually she encouraged John to stand up to his father, while making it clear to his father that John was plenty man enough for her. As his confidence increased he ceased to experience erectile failure.

Dominant, humiliating or suffocating parents quite often contribute to erectile difficulty, especially in younger men. Performance is associated with fear of punishment of one sort or another, and fear, as we've seen, is a powerful inhibitor.

Relationships are sometimes stuck in interaction that looks, to the outsider at least, very unsatisfactory. Often the sex life of the couple will have ground to a halt. Restoring a more healthy balance between the couple often allows the sexual aspects to come back. Sometimes, however, a man's impotence may be subtly encouraged by his wife, who does not want him to be more sexually active in case it places demands on her she does not want to meet, or he might find satisfaction elsewhere.

Similarly, a man who has been so overprotected by his parents that no rebellion is possible, may find that if his partner is at all demanding or there is conflict in the relationship, he doesn't know how to handle it. He may become impotent or avoid sex altogether if he isn't able to learn a way of handling conflict. Sometimes the withholding of sex is the most negative action he can allow in the relationship, and the payoff is that he does not set himself up for failure again in losing his erection.

In a relationship that has been good, a sudden episode of erectile failure may shake the foundations of the marriage, as this next case shows.

Richard and Peggy, a married couple in their forties, were good companions and their sex life was slightly humdrum but satisfactory. Then one night Richard lost his erection just as they were about to have intercourse. Peggy, disappointed, was reassuring none the less and they did not attach a great deal of importance to the episode. Then it happened again. Richard, at Peggy's insistence, went to his GP and had some tests done. Nothing showed up.

Peggy was more upset than Richard, who had taken it in his stride. He knew that he had become very tired after an extra work overload and that he should take a holiday, but it was difficult to arrange. They tried to have intercourse several times after this, but Richard was so affected by Peggy's concern and worry about him that he was unable to get an erection. He knew the plumbing was still working, because he had night-time erections and could masturbate. His GP referred them to a sex-therapy clinic, where they learned to relax and enjoy the sensual side of their relationship without attempting intercourse. They also took a much-needed holiday. It wasn't long before their sex life was restored, and there was a plus, which was that they had been able to talk about their sex life, obtain fresh information and take more permission to enjoy themselves without fear of failure. Peggy, in particular, was encouraged to relax and take care of her own sexual needs from time to time. No longer humdrum or routine, their sex life blossomed. Had they not had this help, it might have been a very different story.

Lack of information and ignorance about sexual function can contribute greatly to sexual problems of every description. Clear, accurate information is given to people attending sex-therapy clinics, and it is often invaluable. There is also a lack of embarrassment which is refreshing, and the people attending the clinic know that once discharged they will never meet their therapist again. This tight, professional boundary is invaluable, as it enables people to feel safe enough to work intensively in this most intimate and private area of our lives. Neither will they be judged or criticized for their sexual conduct. There is one proviso: as with nearly all agencies, anyone stepping over legal boundaries in their sexual life cannot expect this to be confidential, if the safety or welfare of others is at risk.

Robert was newly married and enjoying a good sexual relationship with his wife, who was open-minded. Robert himself was unsure about part of his sexual behaviour and wanted to check with someone that it was all right to behave as he did. His partner did not have a problem with it. Robert's main trigger for excitement and arousal was shoes, ideally black or red ones with high spike heels and pointed toes. He liked his partner to put them on and walk all over him while she wore them. He found it difficult to get an erection without these objects being involved. Assessment revealed that at four years of age his twin sister had been killed in a traffic accident. He had been standing next to her at the time. His shocked mother, who worked in a shoe factory and always wore high heels, stood at the door as he clung to her feet, trying to tell her what had happened. Somehow he had clung to shoes and feet as symbols of what he needed to function. Later they became associated with sexual excitement. It was harmless activity and his wife was generous in joining in with his fantasy. Eventually he lost his impotence in other situations as his confidence increased and he no longer needed the shoes every time they had sex. His sexual behaviour was not illegal, nor did it involve unwilling participants; his partner, though a little puzzled, loved him enough to accept that this was part of his sexual world, and did not try to make him feel bad about it. Some understanding of his need for these objects was helpful to him, as it was to his wife.

Everyone has their own conditions for good sex. What do you need? Look at the list below and see if these conditions are necessary to you:

- a warm comfortable place that is private;
- feeling relaxed with your partner;
- feeling anticipatory excitement and arousal;
- not overtired or stressed;
- plenty of time if you need it (quickies can be fun!);
- no interruptions – turn off that mobile phone!
- clear signals from your partner regarding sexual activity;
- knowing what you like and asking for it;
- feeling physically comfortable;
- relaxed interaction with partner in the preceding hours;
- a partner participating fully in love-making who lets her needs be known and takes responsibility for her own arousal.

This is a fairly typical list for many people, but others may vary in what they require.

Their list might include:

- dressing up;
- fantasy, pornographic, or erotic material;
- physical pain and chastisement;
- bondage games;
- a risk of being seen;
- drugs such as amyl nitrate or cocaine;
- threesomes and multiple partners;
- use of sex aids, telephone sex, prostitutes.

Sex therapists will take these aspects in their stride, and make a decision about whether, and how, they can work with the couple. Outside their remit is a further group of people who cannot have satisfactory sex without involving illegal activities, which include:

- illegal involvement of children or animals;
- sexual violence;
- child pornography;
- voyeurism;
- public masturbation.

There are clinics that deal with these folk, but they are more likely to be under a forensic heading, and not the province of the general sex therapist. Often clients attend because the law requires them to. Issues to do with power and control are often more of an issue than the sex itself.

Dysfunctional men who commit crimes of rape, for example, are excited by the fear they instil, as well as the control and power they have. They are quite frequently impotent and unable to ejaculate while with their victim. The average man who is impotent with his partner is not one of these, needless to say.

Many couples require some of the conditions of the first list, but also one or two from the second list, as the case of Robert and his wife illustrates. If your sex life has become a bit humdrum and you think some excitement is needed, try to vary what you do, where you do it and how you do it. The hard bit is taking your partner along with you in this, especially if you have been impotent and now are not, and she has gone off it. Gentleness and wooing, that old-fashioned courtship technique, will often work wonders with an older woman.

Sometimes a man can become fixated on a sexual activity he feels would greatly excite him, but his partner is not keen. Oral or anal sex is a case in point. If a man becomes impotent, he may think that the answer lies in having more exciting activity with his partner, or outside his marriage. This may be partly true, and shy hesitant partners may need enticing into more adventurous sex, provided they are not coerced into doing something they profoundly disagree with or find painful or repulsive – if this is the case, their partner will have to accept it. Some men are impotent with their wives but not with girlfriends or prostitutes (and vice versa), and this can be because their wives have lost interest or are rather inhibited sexually. It is, of course, also true that younger women are often seen as more attractive, and there is the additional thrill of the forbidden when the woman is a prostitute or part of an extra-marital relationship. However, the majority of people, in studies that have been done, claim that the best sex they have is with their partner in a committed relationship, because of the confidence and sense of security and familiarity with their partner. Whether men who have been impotent within their marriage and are now in a new relationship continue to experience this improvement once their new relationship has become established, is hard to say. I feel doubtful about it myself.

There will be couples who have been through the sex therapy programme, and for whom it has worked in terms of the man regaining his erections, but the female partner has then lost interest sexually in the whole subject. It's fine to want what you can't have, but when it's provided you then have to think about why you wanted it and whether it was really what you wanted after all. The view of a marriage as a system is a valid one. Partners can and do change sides. She wants him to be sexual, because she's highly sexed, but he's not. He becomes sexual, and she promptly goes off it. What's going on here? Couples operate a system of projections between them, in which, in a well-balanced relationship, each will have a fair share of attributes. When things become extreme, and partners become polarized, one is generally expressing something for the other partner. If she complained that he was impotent and therefore deficient as a partner, and he becomes fully functional, how will she express her anger? What has happened here? It's likely that she is holding on to some real anger with him which is not to do with sex, but to do with all sorts of other issues, like feeling trapped, second best, unhappy, unconfident in her own sexuality. Sort out one bit and another bit needs dealing with. If you are in such a relationship, you may want to battle it out between you, which will work if you are prepared to be honest and listen to your partner, but you may want to use a third party to help you sort it out.

7
What to do about it

We've seen how a lack of confidence can play a part in erectile problems. Restoring self-confidence is important, whether the impotence persists or not, and your partner's assistance in this is crucial, especially when she might be feeling upset or unable to understand the need to remain relaxed about it. This is why the lack of confidence becomes a shared problem, and why sex therapy is attempted with couples, rather than just one partner. Therapy aside, there is a great deal you can do to help the situation yourself.

Permission

Give yourself permission *not* to focus on performance. Maybe it will happen, maybe it won't. Erections are like the proverbial Number Nine Bus: if you miss one, there's another one coming along in a little while. Be patient. What do you have to prove? Who to? Are you your own fiercest critic? If you are, let yourself off the hook.

Be assertive

If your partner makes you feel small and unhappy, and it's contributing to your impotence, tell her how you feel and ask her to stop. Don't get angry about it, just say it normally: 'I feel about so high when you talk to me like that. It doesn't help me to feel better about things. I'd really like you to start showing me some appreciation and support instead. I'd value that very much, because I want us to be okay together, more than anything.' If you state your own true feelings assertively, you may be surprised at the outcome. It's unlikely that your partner will listen and not respond, so you'll need to take a deep breath and think about responding to her feelings. She may be quite shocked and upset, and need some reassurance, but she'll remember what you said. To women who have partners who are not assertive or able to push their own point of view in the relationship, my advice is to back off and encourage them to come forward to meet you halfway. Is he afraid of upsetting you? Afraid of displeasing you? Do you like this situation? Let him know it makes you unhappy, that you're not made of glass; that you'd appreciate him being a bit more proactive and taking charge from time to time, even if it means challenging you. Let him know you appreciate him and why. Give yourselves permission to change.

Relax

The conditions for good sex do not usually include being wound up, tense and anxious. Excitement is different. Think about ways in which you can relax.

Start pampering yourself. Lie in a warm scented bath with a glass of something refreshing, and relax. Perhaps it does sound girly, but what's wrong with that? Have some music playing nearby. Is there anything else you can add – candles, soft fluffy towels, body lotion? Encourage your partner to do the same when she seems tense or tired.

Try an all-over body rub and massage, using oils or lotion. Offer your partner one. Relaxation techniques include breathing deeply and slowly, and there are plenty of tapes that will give you instructions about this. Deep relaxation is very good for you; it lowers your blood pressure and pulse rate and helps you feel calm and peaceful. After a stressful day in the office in a competitive working environment, with a difficult journey either side and a late supper when you get home at seven, your body will be in need of some care and nurture at the end of the day. Work is sometimes good for our wallet but not for our health. Exercise is good for releasing tension and making you feel better, and if you can follow this at bedtime with a relaxation session, so much the better. If you don't enjoy exercise, you might consider buying a dog, which gives you a reason to go out for a walk and is in itself a stress reducer. Having a furry or hairy animal to stroke is soothing anyway, and it seems as if humans have a deep need for physical touch, almost a grooming instinct, if they can recognize it. Fatigue and stress are common components of a working life these days, and impotence can follow on from this. We all need a certain amount of stress in order to function, but when there's a systems overload, the body

59

shuts down certain functions. We stop sleeping and don't wake feeling refreshed if we do sleep, or we sleep all the time; we become angry at the drop of a hat; we start to drink more than we did; we don't talk to our partners; we may develop high blood pressure; we forget things; we lose our desire for sex, and impotence begins to be a feature when we try to have sex and our body doesn't want to co-operate. Pretty soon we can be depressed and burned out. It's very important to turn this around, and if you're in a job that is demanding and stressful, or there are other changes in your life as well, look after your body and your relationship and be aware of the warning signs. Where both parties are in demanding jobs there is a temptation to avoid sex or real intimacy because there's no time for it.

Put your embarrassment to one side

Supposing you're under quite a lot of stress and one more thing happens to knock you down. You begin to feel swamped, and to cap it all you can't get an erection. You don't have any energy for desire anyway, but it panics you that this normal function should suddenly have stopped. Should you go and see your doctor? Probably, especially if you are not having any erections at all, despite attempting to arouse yourself via magazines, etc. If you have a health problem, the sooner it's diagnosed the better. If you don't, then taking care of yourself and maybe making some life changes will be helpful. Overcome your embarrassment and go back to your doctor, and ask for a referral to a sex-therapy clinic. Keep talking to your partner; she will be concerned about you, but it may not appear that way at times, as she may become frustrated and want you to sort it out on your own.

8
Sex therapy

What happens when you visit a sex therapist? Let me make one thing clear from the outset – nothing happens in the therapy sessions besides talking, thinking and sharing information. No undressing or demonstrations of the problem. The therapist knows how to work with you to reach the most accurate assessment. There are generally more female than male therapists of every type, but the proportion of males to females is slightly higher in psychosexual therapy. I mention this because it seems important that in this very personal and intimate area, men should have a choice, if possible, about the gender of their therapist. You may, however, be referred by your GP to the clinic your doctor has a link with, but you can always phone to ask if there is a male therapist available there, if you wish. If you have a strong preference for a man and there isn't one available, you may consider looking at the BASRT website and finding a male therapist in private practice.

In the larger clinics there may be medical staff in addition to the therapist, who will carry out any medical tests required in order to make a thorough assessment. Relate and private practices refer their clients to a doctor they have an agreement with, or the client's own GP, for these tests, if they are needed; they do not carry them out themselves.

First you will be sent an appointment, for yourself and your partner to attend. If you do not want your partner to attend with you, you can attend on your own and discuss this with the therapist. They will tell you whether, and why, they can or cannot take you on for a sex-therapy programme, and if not, what they can offer you. Having no available partner to attend for sex therapy with you may well be a problem if you intend to become potent again with a partner, as it will indicate difficulties in trust and communication which will need to be resolved before you can begin the treatment programme. If you and your partner are really not getting along, which may or may not be to do with the sexual problem, the sex therapist may well suggest you have some relationship counselling first. They may offer this themselves, but it is more likely they will refer you to a colleague who specializes in this, and then take you both back for a treatment programme once some of the problems have been dealt with.

In this first meeting you will be wondering if you can trust this person, feel confidence in them and be treated with respect as an individual. If you don't, go elsewhere.

Assessment

After this initial meeting with both partners, the Relate sex therapist may well suggest that the assessment continue by offering you individual interviews. (Other psychosexual therapists may work slightly differently.) This is because these assessments are lengthy and take time to complete. From these two assessments the therapist will make a diagnosis and tailor a treatment programme to suit your needs. Sometimes secrets are revealed in these individual sessions that the therapist has to discuss with the person in order to see whether keeping this secret will get in the way of treatment. If the secret is a serious one and will prevent the treatment programme succeeding, the therapist will not offer to continue with the treatment programme. The confidentiality of the partner with the secret is never broken, unless others are at serious risk. Usually where there is a secret, such as an extra-marital affair in the past that the other doesn't know about, the therapist and their client will discuss what, if anything, needs to happen because of it. Sometimes secrets are better left secret. Following the individual assessment meetings, the couple will be invited back to hear the observations and proposals of the therapist regarding their sexual relationship and the problem they came with. Most therapists like to do this all-round evaluation of their clients, and in my experience a good thorough evaluation, shared with the couple, enables them to understand why the problem has occurred, what led up to it, what is keeping it in place and, very importantly, what the therapist feels is a way forward. If the assessment has uncovered serious difficulties in the relationship which would prevent treatment from succeeding, the couple will be told about this honestly and helped to sort this out before treatment can begin. Adjustments will happen in the relationship anyway if the treatment plan is followed, but if the relationship is basically sound this will not create too much of a problem.

Treatment programmes: homework

The next step is for the therapist to begin the treatment programme by giving homework assignments. The homework assignments take place at home, in the privacy of your own bedroom or other chosen place, and the co-operation of partners is vital. Each week you will be able to say how it went, what happened and what it felt like. This is often very encouraging. Then you will be given the next assignment. The purpose of the assignments, which I will not describe in detail, is to enable a couple to create some private, good quality time and space on a regular basis for themselves, and to start from the beginning again to relearn, without any pressure, a satisfying sexual interaction. Specific techniques are taught, and information given, which is helpful and interesting. As any couple in sex therapy are learning the delights of the sexual menu by starting with the aperitifs and appetizers, and creating the optimum conditions to partake in these, they will be instructed not to go on to the main course too soon. Not, in fact, until the therapist gives them permission. It's so easy to sabotage something, even accidentally, by jumping the gun, that this instruction must be heeded.

Gradually the confidence of both partners will return. Negative ideas, thoughts and feelings will be ironed out, and the couple will function sexually once more in a way that is more relaxed, forgiving and sexually fulfilling. Once the man is getting regular erections again with the help of his partner, and is able to lose and regain them without anxiety, the couple will be encouraged to move towards penetration, with his erect penis quietly inside her vagina for a short while. Re-stimulating the penis if the erection goes off a bit is encouraged, but the need for him to 'perform' is ruled out. As each step is managed and given encouragement, they will gradually move forward to more active intercourse.

If something is fundamentally very much amiss in the relationship, and it then comes to light during these homework sessions, the therapist may want to take some time out from therapy to work on this, before proceeding. In my experience, there is always a point mid-way through the process when things wobble. The man wants to be instantly cured and can't see the point of all this faffing around in the bedroom without getting and using his erection. The female may be sick and tired of the whole process, which may seem mechanical and as if all the attention is on the man. Both may lose heart with each other and the whole process. Some real anger and resentment may surface at this point, with one another and the therapist. Therapists understand this (maddeningly!) and are trained to enable couples to take responsibility for what is happening, look at it, work with it and move on. The success rates for couples who do stick with it are high.

For men and their partners where there is an organic reason for loss of erection from time to time, a programme tailored to their needs will help them to maximize what they have, and encourage them to vary their approach, adding in other helpful strategies as and when. This might include Viagra, or some helpful prosthetic device.

Of course, for men wanting instant solutions, sex therapy is not going to seem very attractive – more like hard work. And it may be expensive, unless NHS funded. My response to that is: if my car breaks down I want someone skilled and experienced in the art of fixing cars, someone who will tell me honestly what the problem is. Maybe I know the fault is due to engine wear and a flat tyre, but knowing it doesn't fix the car. Having someone to confirm what I thought and offer me a way to get the car running again is much more helpful. I've still got to take it to the garage, but that's the first step to getting it fixed.

Sex therapists do not have a shortage of clients, neither do they like to waste their time or yours. If they feel they can't help you, they'll say so. If they and you want to give it a go and it doesn't work, as sometimes happens, it may be because the therapist was persuaded against their own better judgement to offer treatment, or you or your partner held back something vital to the process. Generally it's a very successful form of treatment, but there are no guarantees.

Sex therapy is a behavioural approach: that is, it is task centred. As the sessions proceed, the therapist will give positive feedback on the homework assignments. Restoring confidence is at the heart of the work, and any couple who have experienced disappointment and sexual frustration will need the positive encouragement and support of the therapist to give them a boost, even when things don't go well. Gradually, as the man's erections return and his partner too gains in confidence, the therapy sessions will wind down, but there is rarely an abrupt cut-off point, and most clinics offer follow-up appointments three months after therapy has finished. One aim of the therapist will be to ensure the couple know what to do if the problems should recur. This in itself gives confidence to the couple, who now have control over their lives in a way that was not possible before. What we learn about and know can be put aside all too quickly when we are feeling angry, upset and disappointed, but if both partners have had the learning one can pull the other out of despondency by reminding them of what they need to do to make it work again.

After the initial nervousness of the first meeting, in my experience there is sometimes a great deal of warmth and humour in subsequent sessions with couples. This is because the sexual part of our lives is linked to the excitement and thrill of adolescence, which is re-awakened in the therapy. The couple who have been accepted for treatment generally have a good enough relationship, or they would not be there. Adding the sexual component makes it something really special. No wonder there is sometimes laughter in the room.

9

Other factors

Women go off sex from time to time too. They become exhausted from lack of sleep when their babies are tiny. They feel washed out by excessive blood loss if they have heavy periods, and are sometimes depressed and exhausted by menopausal symptoms. Their sexual appetites may be flattened by years of taking the contraceptive pill. They may have had years of caring for children, elderly parents, house and husband as well as working outside the home. Enthusiasm and energy for sex can be severely depleted in these situations, and if you add to this a significant loss of some description, such as the death of a parent, it's not hard to see that the same situations that can lead to male impotence are present for women too. Women will put up with sex, even though they may not enjoy it. This is not pleasant for their husbands, if they know, but they may not know that their wife is not enjoying it. Women can fake sexual satisfaction, in a way that is difficult for a man to emulate. His erection is the signal that he is aroused. If he becomes impotent he can't lie about it, his penis is telling a different story. If his wife takes it personally as a criticism of her, this is not his fault.

Eric, 63, didn't feel like sex. He stopped having erections with his partner Pauline and had no interest in masturbation. Pauline, 60, realized that he might be worried about his forthcoming retirement, but he wouldn't talk about it. She tried everything she could think of – sexy underwear, intimate dinners, approaching him directly hoping to seduce him. He still wasn't interested. He stayed up late, drank too much and avoided being with her in the bedroom until she was asleep. She finally asked him outright what the problem was. He was able to tell her it wasn't her, but that he was feeling a bit low these days and had gone off sex. She drew out of him that he was afraid of the future, when he would no longer be at work and they would have to keep each other company all the time. He didn't know how he was going to manage it. Life seemed empty now, and life after retirement even more bleak. Pauline, who had just retired herself, was able to tell him that his feelings were understandable, and that he would need time to get used to being at home. She told him about the new horizons that were opening up for her, and expressed faith in his ability to use his talents in other ways. Reassurance and permission to talk about some of his feelings without being misunderstood helped him to feel more at one with his wife, but his impotence remained. Eventually, with Pauline's gentle prompting, he went to his doctor, who discovered that he had diet-controlled diabetes. This increased his depression, but once he began treatment and started to look after himself more, he felt his health improve. He talked to the practice counsellor about his depression, though he felt a fraud, but to his surprise it helped. He brought his retirement forward a little and began to look forward to giving up the daily grind, though giving up his status, money and power was harder. He began to understand how tired he had become. Pauline, now she understood, was content to wait for this episode of their lives to pass into a different phase.

Eventually they settled sexually for a mixed economy, using his erections when he got them, and employing other methods at other times, including a new vibrator for her, which excited him greatly the first time they used it and almost made it redundant. If Pauline hadn't asked directly what the problem was, and if Eric hadn't answered truthfully, they might have struggled on in a very unhappy marriage for a long time.

Often it seems that people don't know why they feel so low, miserable or fed up. They are in a situation they can't easily change and talking doesn't change anything, they reason.

Actually, talking does change quite a lot. This is how –

Talking can help

- It gets some of the grey foggy mess inside the mind out into the open.
- Once outside, it becomes more visible.
- Once more visible and understandable, it assumes a shape and an identity. It becomes real, not a nebulous set of clogging emotions.
- Moving it from *in here* to *out there* means you make some sense of it as you do it. It unravels like a thread when pulled.

- As it unravels, so do the feelings you have about it.
- Once it's unravelled, out here and in the room, it becomes much easier to decide what to do with it. Bits of it may not belong to you; other people may be responsible for them. Perhaps you can hand them over. Bits of it may need to be examined and then left behind. Bits may need to be stored for future use. Gradually the depressed feeling will become sorted out and made sense of, and some decisions made about what to do, if this is required.

When I've asked depressed people at times what their inner world would look like if they could see it as a room in a building, they have sometimes said, 'There's a load of objects hidden under dust-sheets. I keep stumbling over them,' or 'There are no windows and the light is off. I don't know where the door is.' These images are very revealing, and already the person is becoming aware of the nature of their inner world. The therapist might then help the person to use these images to find a way forward. Dust-sheets can be lifted a little and the hidden object identified, a source of light for the dark room might come from some other person, or the client's own insight. The client and the therapist may have to stay and experience the darkness together and feel their way around the edge. It is, as you can tell, an approach that interests and excites me a great deal, because it worked for me.

If you intend to talk about what's making you depressed, choose a good safe place to do it. Partners may not always understand, or come at the problem from a different angle, proposing solutions to you that aren't yours in their anxiety to see you better. Friends may be more helpful. Your doctor has limited time to listen and may well suggest counselling. Give it a try if it's suggested. What have you got to lose? Is talking really so dangerous? Remember, the person who has control over the talking – how, when, where and who to – is you.

All this has a direct effect upon impotence caused or maintained by depression.

Change

Finally, a word about change. Change involves loss, a transition from one state to another, leaving one behind. Loss generates anger as well as sadness. Nothing stays the same for ever: we grow, we move on, eventually we die. Ageing is changing. We can fight it, cosmetically, in which case we will be sure to lose eventually, despite pouring money into the coffers of Botox manufacturers and cosmetic surgeons. We may decide it's worth it for the short-term gain. Or we can go with it, riding the wave as it were. If you have become impotent through some irreversible medical condition, you can decide to accept celibacy and make the most of it, or you can take advantage of what technology or the drug industry has to offer. Celibacy has its own rewards: no need to prove anything, fewer distractions, relationships based on a different premise. A relationship without penetrative sexual intercourse does not have to exclude sex altogether. There are many ways to give a partner sexual and sensual satisfaction, and if you as the male feel uninterested because you can't personally face offering something you can't partake of yourself, ask yourself whether you really believe that for good sex you absolutely have to have an erection and maintain it. What would your partner say to that? Good sex for her may depend on very different things. Many women find that they are sexually aroused in situations where penetration is not possible, such as in a public place. Many find that if their partner offers them all over caressing, with oral or manual stimulation of the area around their clitoris, with the optional use of a vibrator, they achieve intense orgasms with their partners. Yet no erection is necessary. Numerous intermittently impotent men I have known have tried this process of courtship and love-making with their partners, and have found that kissing, caressing, stroking, undressing, and gentle love-making has so excited their partner that they too have become aroused. But if it doesn't happen, you've had the satisfaction of giving your partner a really good time. Maybe women are less impressed by the size, hardness and thrust of a man's penis than men think they are. It's a matter of context.

Ejaculation is what provides the man with sexual release, and the ability to ejaculate can be impaired by prostate surgery, for example, where ejaculation may take place, but internally. For men with impaired circulation and damage to the blood vessels of the penis, the use of whatever assistance is recommended by your clinic should ensure you ejaculate as before. Like drawing water from a well, the hydraulic system may need repair, but the water stays the same. I would say to couples who have had a previously good sex life now interrupted by impotence, '*Continue to make love, in whatever way you choose. Forget about him getting an erection, immerse yourself in the pleasure of your partner, and incorporate any help you require into your love-making as you need it. And keep talking.*'

Celibacy

Celibacy, as I said before, is also a real option. Couples who opt for this may struggle with affectionate intimacy in case they feel sexual arousal, which can stir the old feelings of disappointment and loss. If this can be resolved, the non-sexual affection still existing between them will show in the small warm gestures and physical closeness of the couple in a way that is very comforting. Throughout the ages some men and women have chosen the path of celibacy deliberately, believing it would lead to a higher understanding and acceptance, or enlightenment, or spirituality. It is a choice, for impotent men and others.

Making the best of sex

For other more sexually interested horny little devils, there are the gizmos and gadgets mentioned in a previous chapter. And how many men can have an erection to order, anyway? You can, if you're using one of these, provided you have a partner happy to take part. This is really the crux of the matter.

An older man who becomes impotent may well have a wife who is not too well, or who, since the menopause, has found intercourse difficult and not very enjoyable, because of vaginal dryness or other difficulty. The couple may decide to call it a day, sexually. Their sexual feelings may well be diminished but they will rarely vanish entirely. Like an underground stream, sexuality will bubble up in different ways and have to be diverted. Masturbation may be an answer, and it's good for both sexes in keeping the sexual organs healthy. Of course, it has to be at an appropriate time and place, but there should be no shame attached to it. An older man, unable to have sex with his wife, may find himself becoming over-interested in young women around him. This is upsetting for his wife quite often, and may well be upsetting for the man, not to mention the young women, but denied sexual feelings are hard to contain all the time. Perhaps society needs to be more understanding about this, as it's often the physical closeness he wants to regain, rather than a full-blown sexual relationship. Of course, children and young people need to be protected from these advances, if they get out of hand, and we need to teach our young people how to assertively put back these boundaries. Partners not offering sex to their partner are sometimes afraid that offering affection instead will be misread as a demand for sex. It helps to know, verbally, what the situation is, and if affection is offered the couple may function much more happily.

10

Bringing back the sparkle

In this chapter, we will look at ways of making a sex life that has become disappointing and mundane, because of impotence or depression, more loving and exciting. If you have lost heart, or you're bored, or uninterested in sex, there are some things you can do to bring back the twinkle in your eye.

- Notice what your partner does that is positive and respond positively. Whether it's making a cup of tea for you, remembering a family birthday or remaining outwardly calm when you're backing into a small parking place – give it a positive comment. It has to be genuine and accurate. Of course, you may need to give some negative feedback too, but a ratio of three positives to one negative is good. It restores confidence as nothing else.
- Try not to nag, bear grudges or worry about things – it distracts from any sexual or sensual pleasure you might otherwise be enjoying, and it's also a distraction from any other pleasant interactions your life might contain. If you are a born worrier and go over past grievances a great deal, you might need help to deal with these, but getting involved in an activity that involves other people can take your mind off other worries of your own. For most of the negative stuff that happens in our lives, involving deaths and accidents, there's not a lot we can do about any of it anyway. Shit happens, as they say, but while it isn't happening we can enjoy and be thankful for what we have now.
- Before you criticize your spouse, think about what you want to say. Feedback should be constructive, clear and honest, rather than an outright attack. It should contain what you would like to happen, as well as what went wrong. If communication between you improves because you have put some effort into it, I can guarantee your sex life will also improve.
- Keep yourself in good shape. Dress up a bit when you go out with your partner. A decent hair cut for an older man is worth spending money on. Feel good about yourself and your confidence will increase.

- Take up an activity that you both enjoy – dancing is good, so is horse riding, swimming or tennis, for example. Even if you're not sure you'd enjoy salsa dancing, say, or pub quizzes, give it a try. You might surprise yourself!
- Make your bedroom a place of comfort, relaxation and erotic pleasure. Soft lights, a bed the right height for you, pillows and a music system all help. Aromatherapy oils and a burner appeal to some people, as well as fresh flowers, some chilled wine – spend time thinking about these things. Re-decorate if the room is dowdy or not to your taste.
- Find small ways to please your partner – flowers, magazines, outings – whatever they like. It doesn't have to cost the earth.
- Some couples have the equivalent of a Chinese pillow-book – a book of erotic or sensuous images. We are not talking about hard porn here, but erotica. There are many erotic novels for women, for instance, which are readily available and arousing for women. There are no pictures, only erotic fantasy.
- Clothing that is sensuous to touch – silk, satin, lace – gives added allure. Costume dramas often depend on understated sexuality, and it's very potent. (Think about Mr Darcy in wet shirt and breeches.) Young women often wear very flimsy minimal clothing when they go out, but older women may grow to appreciate the sexual allure of the barely glimpsed lace undergarment. The hidden attraction is sometimes more interesting than the goods on full display.
- Find out what you like. Experiment a bit. Take it in turns to ask your partner what they would like. Try it, even if it doesn't appeal to you. If you both think it might be fun, and it doesn't harm anybody else, go ahead. Some people find variations such as anal sex exciting; for others it's painful. Oral sex can be viewed as highly arousing (it is for most men), but there are women who do not enjoy this. If you try something and don't enjoy it, try something else – fur, feathers, silk scarves, handcuffs, fancy condoms – there's a huge menu once you start looking.
- Listen to your partner. If you are a man who has experienced an episode of impotence, you may have some ground to make up with your partner. What has been going on in her life all the time you have been worrying about your willy? Unspoken fears, worries and anxieties clog up our emotional and cognitive

processes and get in the way of our relationships. Negative stuff is hard to say sometimes, but it still needs saying, gently and honestly. If you have been waiting every evening for her to go to bed and sleep so that you do not have to try to have sex with her, she will be hurt and upset. If she has made an effort to seduce you and please you and you have ignored her, she will also be hurt and upset. This is because she feels she has probably lost your affection too, and she doesn't understand what's going on. Tell her.

- Put the affection back. It's likely she's been starved of it and will be feeling unloved and resentful. There's a difference between affection and sex; often if one goes, so does the other. There's an automatic association in the minds of many people that if you demonstrate or receive affection you will be expected to have a sexual encounter with that person. Many women, feeling sexually disappointed, back away from this. A kiss, a hug, a stroke of the arm, an arm round the shoulder costs nothing and does not indicate immediate sexual action to follow. Feeling unloved because the partner who used to kiss and hold you does not do that any more is worse for many women than not having sex with him because he is indisposed. Signals have to be clear, and intentions have to be stated if we're unsure.

- Acknowledge the loss. The loss of your sexual function is not just your loss, it's also your partner's loss. For a while she has lost the person she knew, felt unhappy and confused about what was going on and may have felt unloved and distant from you. It's something you share, just as you can share the rebuilding and revitalizing of your sexual life together in whatever form it now takes.

- It takes a while to recover from a change in our circumstances, when it affects us so deeply. You and your partner may be at different places along this path. Talking will help, affection will help, patience and understanding will help.

Overall, I'm a great believer in marriage; it's never perfect but it's often the best there is, and I know it's hard work. Often the emotional work of the marriage falls to the female partner. Many men, who view their main role as provider for their family and head of their household, may not understand that to keep their marriage stable and solid something more is needed from them – the ability to be honest with their partner. This is especially the case if they experience erectile failure. It's then that their confidence becomes really shaky, and if they haven't had an open honest relationship with their wife or partner up to that point, it's hard to start now. A wife who doesn't understand how difficult this can be for her husband may become frustrated and angry with him. She may not want to hear how tired, depressed or fed up he is. This is where the hard work of marriage happens; either they take stock and listen to one another or things fail even more. We're talking about being open about feelings here, not about attacking the other partner; it can be done, but it often feels risky.

Marco was unable to get an erection after he had an operation for bowel cancer, followed by further surgery in the form of a heart bypass. The nerves to his genitals had been damaged during the surgery. He felt physically better than he had before the operation, but mourned the loss of his sexual life. His wife understood he missed this keenly, though she wasn't too worried about it for herself. She had nearly lost him; he had lost his sexual potency and his work prospects. Both had things to grieve for and recover from. Once they had been through a period of mourning and the changes in their lives had been processed, they began to look at what was left to them regarding their sex life. They found their doctor very understanding, and were referred to a clinic where they were helped to decide on a suitable form of treatment. Although Marco knows he may not have long to live, especially if the cancer comes back, he's too intent on enjoying the life he has to worry overmuch about what he cannot change. Selina, his wife, has learned not to live in constant terror of him collapsing when they do make love (and it is a possibility), and has adopted a fatalistic approach. For them, the important thing is that they are still together and can still enjoy a natural, if assisted, sex life together.

Conclusion

As we've seen, impotence can be a complex condition. It touches on the deeply personal and intimate parts of a person's life with their partner. It involves not just the plumbing, which may or may not be faulty, but also the man's perception of himself, his partner and his life. Take heart. You are not alone. What's more, there are people out there willing to share their experience of erectile dysfunction and how they dealt with it. However, you may need to hold on to your reservations about sex therapy and give it a try. If you do, the chances of a successful outcome are high. The drawback is that you may be asked to discuss aspects of your life you would rather not think about, much less discuss. Courage is needed here, and you may not want to go down that road.

If you can be offered some other treatment, and if confidence is at the core of the problem, a medical solution such as Viagra, if you have a partner to use it with, might provide a way of regaining your confidence and potency. Cognitive therapy can also be helpful, as it stops the thought about failure from taking hold and turns it into a positive thought. It's not always easy to find cognitive behavioural therapists, however.

If there is a purely medical reason for your impotence, and your relationship is good, there are several different avenues open to you. You do need a thorough assessment to make sure you receive the right help, and your partner will need to get involved. Remember, changes to our health, like changes to our marital status, social or economic status, all involve loss, and this requires adjustment. Loss generates anger, which needs some working through.

Most episodes of impotence pass in time anyway, when there is no organic cause, and they usually pass when the man feels less depressed or overloaded or tired.

If there is good communication between the spouses and no pressure is put on the man to perform, this will usually happen sooner rather than later. A man who knows that his impotence is the result of his being overloaded in some way is more likely to forgive himself and give himself time to recover. If his partner gets anxious and worries about him not loving her any more and he offers no reassurance to her, she may well become very despondent, whereas if she understands that this is a temporary state of affairs she is more likely to sit it out and be supportive. Lack of support can show itself in many ways. Not touching is the most obvious signal that something is wrong. You can do something about this, and you need to.

It does a lot of good sometimes to stop still and take stock of the situation. Sex therapy can offer you this space and time, enclosed in its own private place, in which to consider and get to know what your impotence is all about, and how to manage it. Being involved in this with your partner is, I believe, an activity which really can enhance the life of the couple, and I don't just mean sexually.

Even if you're impotent and depressed and do nothing about it, you may feel better after a time, but if your partner has lost interest and you have stopped talking to her about it (or maybe have never talked to her about it), a dead or ended marriage will not improve your impotence or your confidence in yourself, even if the cause of the problem was partly your partner's treatment of you. This is why it is such a shared problem, and often such a complex one. The good news is that with both of you in tune and being honest with one another, there is much that you can do to help yourselves, and there is a great deal of good reliable help out there to assist you. What's more, it's becoming increasingly acceptable to make use of it, in the way in which we seek assistance for other problems. Don't be shy, step forward and take the first step to improving your love life – together.

Bibliography

Fulghum Bruce, Debra
The Unofficial Guide to Conquering Impotence, Wiley 1999
ISBN 0-02862-870-5

Carrol, Dr Steve
The Which? Guide to Men's Health, Which? Consumer Guides 1999
ISBN 0-85202-758-3

Katzenstein, Larry
Viagra: The Potency Promise, St Martin's Paperbacks 1998
ISBN 0-31296-929-5

Kell, Philip, and Dinsmore, Wallace
Impotence: A Guide for Men of All Ages, Royal Society of Medicine
Press 2002
ISBN 1-85315-402-4

Milsten, Richard, and Slowinski, Julian
The Sexual Male: Problems and Solutions, W.W. Norton 2000
ISBN 0-39332-127-4

Rowe, Dorothy
Depression: The Way Out of Your Prison, Brunner Routledge 1996
ISBN 0-41514-482-5

Zilbergeld, Bernard
Men and Sex, HarperCollins 1995
ISBN 0-00638-323-8

Useful addresses

Addresses and websites

Impotence Association
PO Box 10296
London
SW17 9WH
Helpline 020 8767 7791
www.impotence.org.uk

The Impotence Association and The Men's Health Forum
Tel. 0870 129 0100
www.informed.org.uk

Porterbrook Clinic (NHS psychosexual clinic)
www.porterbrookclinic.com

National Kidney and Urologic Diseases Information Clearing House
www.niddk.nih.gov

Supporting agencies and clinics

ACCORD Marriage Care (previously Catholic Marriage Advisory Centre, Northern Ireland)
Cana House
56 Lisburn Road
Belfast
BT9 6AF
Tel. 028 90 233 002

British Association for Counselling and Psychotherapy (BACP)
1 Regent Place
Rugby
CV21 2PJ
Tel. 0870 4435252

British Association for Sexual and Relationship Therapy (BASRT)
PO Box 13686
London
SW20 9ZH
www.basrt.org.uk (includes lists of psychosexual practitioners and clinics)

Couple Counselling Scotland
18 York Place
Edinburgh
EH1 3EP
Tel. 0131 558 9669
www.couplecounselling.org

Diabetes UK
10 Park Way
London
NW1 7AA
Careline 020 7420 1030 (voice) 020 7424 1888 (text)
www.diabetes.org.uk

Institute of Psychosexual Medicine
12 Chandos Street
Cavendish Square
London
W1G 9DR
Tel. 020 7580 0631
www.ipm.org.uk

Jewish Marriage Council
23 Ravenshurst Avenue
London
NW4 4EE
Tel. 020 8203 8311

Marriage Care
Clitherow House
1 Blythe Mews
Blythe Road
London
W14 0NW
Helpline 0845 757 3921

Relate (English headquarters)
Herbert Gray College
Little Church Street
Rugby
CV21 3AP
Helpline 0845 130 40 10
Tel. 01788 573 241 (local numbers in phone book for psychosexual
and marital therapy appointments)
www.relate.org

Relate (Northern Ireland)
74–76 Dublin Road
Belfast
BT2 7HP
Tel. 028 90 323 454

SPOD (Association to Aid the Sexual and Personal Relationships of
People with a Disability)
286 Camden Road
London
N7 0BJ
Tel. 020 7607 8851

Index